Stop The BS!

Stop The BS!

I Just Want The Truth About Dieting, Supplements, Weight Loss, and Exercise.

Lewis Meline, M.D.

ISBN: Softcover 978-0-9979155-4-9
eBook 978-0-9979115-5-6

Rev. date: 03/24/2018

To order additional copies of this book, contact:
Dr. Meline by email: DrMeline@SS-Health.com, or visit www.SS-Health.com

CONTENTS

INTRODUCTION

THIS BOOK WAS WRITTEN TO DISPEL THE FALLACIES that are being perpetuated about diets, supplements, weight loss, and exercise. The **MULTITUDE** of weight-loss programs and supplements have developed into a **MULTIBILLION**-dollar industry with **NO IMPACT ON WEIGHT LOSS and WITHOUT ANY IMPROVEMENT IN OVERALL HEALTH.** This includes books and programs developed by prominent television physicians and personalities, research by the medical community, and new medications.

OBESITY is now considered a **MAJOR HEALTH PROBLEM**, and much research is being performed to determine the cause and ways to treat it. **NUTRITIONAL HEALTH** has also been on the decline despite the enormous number of supplements and nutritional aids in the form of herbs and natural medicines.

It's **AMAZING** that **RESEARCH** and all these **PROGRAMS** and **SUPPLEMENTS** have **FAILED** to address the most basic cause of obesity. Also, the **DIET PROGRAMS** and **SUPPLEMENTS** are **NOT EFFECTIVE** because they **ARE ALL FALLACIES**. They make bold claims but deliver nothing.

IF YOU REALLY WANT TO KNOW THE TRUTH ABOUT WEIGHT LOSS AND GOOD HEALTH, READ ON. I know that a lot of books and websites claim to have the truth about these subjects. Why is my book any different? It's because **I DO NOT HAVE AN AGENDA.** There is no program or product to sell. I will clarify information that is available to everyone but is being **MISREPRESENTED and SUPPRESSED** by all the various diet programs and supplement providers.

NEW INFORMATION NOT AVAILABLE ANYWHERE ELSE will also be presented.

BY READING AND HEEDING the information in this book, you WILL be able to achieve your **DESIRED BODY WEIGHT** and **BE HEALTHY** at the same time **WITHOUT** the use of any **SUPPLEMENTS, DIET PROGRAMS, MEDICATIONS,** or other crutches that may be offered to you. You will also be able to maintain your weight and health for a lifetime.

There are no surprise products or gimmicks or hypes, just **HONEST INFORMATION**. You will be surprised at how much you already know but are just being confused by the enormous volume of **MISINFORMATION** that is being thrown at you by various diet programs, supplement promoters, Internet sites, television shows and personalities, high-profile physicians, and the medical community.

Here are a few of the things you will learn as you read this book:

- Why taking a particular supplement or eating one or two special foods will not make you skinny and, in particular, will not make you healthy.
- Why the "natural medicine," fad diets, and other programs are fallacies and designed (whether on purpose or by accident) to move your money from your wallet to theirs.
- There is no such thing as embracing a diet or exercise program or taking a medication for a time and then being able to revert to your old habits that caused the problems in the first place.
- There are **NO** scientific studies that are going to find the magic formula, medication, or diet for weight loss.
- Understand that you will have to make some changes in your lifestyle that will be permanent.
- This information is applicable if you are skinny or fat (including very obese people), healthy or unhealthy, young or old or have medical problems that are physical, psychological, or biochemical in nature.
- What research and all the diet programs and supplements have failed to address—the most basic cause of the problem.
- **Most importantly,** you will understand why people continue to fail at achieving their weight and health goals so you won't fail at yours.

Fortunately, it is **NOT NECESSARY** to have in-depth knowledge or even a superficial knowledge of physiology and nutrition to understand and use the principles necessary for good health. You **DO NOT** have to be well educated or have any particular background to understand the information contained in this book. The facts you need to know are presented in a simple way such that anyone can understand them. I will also be introducing you to *several ideas that are unique* that you will not find discussed anywhere else.

I AM NOT INCLUDING ANY REFERENCES TO SHOW VALIDITY OF THE INFORMATION PRESENTED. This is because I am not presenting new research that needs to be validated. Most of the information is very well-known and easily verified. Just search for the desired topic on Google, and you will find numerous articles confirming what I am telling you in this book. **I WILL JUST BE CLARIFYING THE MISCONCEPTIONS ABOUT THIS KNOWLEDGE.** You will also discover that there will be a lot of detailed information on these websites. This detail just causes confusion as it provides much more information than you need but is not enough to appropriately educate you on the topics discussed.

NO TESTIMONIALS WILL BE USED TO VALIDATE MY INFORMATION. *Using individuals to proclaim validity of a program is meaningless.* Regardless of the supplement, diet program, or psychological profiling that you may encounter, it is easy to find individuals who can use the program and lose weight (or achieve whatever result they are advertising). They are motivated by the promoters to succeed, so it would be unlikely that they would fail. If they did, obviously they would not be included with the testimonials. Also, **MOST TESTIMONIALS ARE FABRICATED**. When you objectively look at the product they are selling and the person giving the testimonial, it is quite obvious that the results could not have been achieved as advertised. (If you have difficulty seeing this now, you will have no problem seeing the fallacy once you have read this book.)

NEW INFORMATION has been obtained from **MANY YEARS OF STUDYING AND USING INFORMATION** from a variety of sources. Many things that I discovered **HAVE NOT BEEN ADDRESSED** by any other source. This is **VERY VALUABLE INFORMATION** that you will need to help you succeed in achieving your ideal weight and health and maintain them for life.

The information in this book *does not* require that you spend any of your money on special food or equipment to support my ideas. The only money that you may spend is to purchase this book, assuming that you cannot borrow it from someone else or check it out from a library. During the time spent reading this book, you will *gain a wealth of knowledge* that will *serve you for a lifetime.* If you are looking for a quick fix to your health and weight problems, do not waste your time with this book—or any other book, diet program, or supplement, for that matter. **IF YOU ARE SERIOUS ABOUT WANTING TO BE HEALTHY AND ACHIEVING AND MAINTAINING A CERTAIN BODY WEIGHT AND HEALTH FOR THE REST OF YOUR LIFE, THIS IS A BOOK YOU MUST READ**.

Reading This Book

Read the information in the order that it is presented. The material builds on itself, so skipping around may lead to some confusion. I also find that most people do not have a good understanding of the material in the first sections. *You need to have a firm understanding of this information before getting into the later sections.* Otherwise, as you apply the ideas that I am presenting, advertisements of dieting programs, supplements, etc., may cause you to do things that will result in failing to achieve your weight and health goals. If you **READ** this book in its **ENTIRETY and USE** the information, you **WILL SUCCEED** in achieving your weight and health goals **WITHOUT THE USE** of supplements, medications, or any other crutches that will be offered to you.

It may be helpful to read some of the material more than once. The principles are simple and straightforward, but there are several things to remember and understand. If you find that some ideas are expressed in different sections, this is not an oversight. I want you to get these ideas firmly entrenched in your mind.

You may already be familiar with some nutrition and physiology. If you are, *still pay attention to the material in the sections that address these topics.* Make sure that you don't have any misconceptions about this information. Many well-educated people have significant misconceptions about nutrition and physiology that can be a huge stumbling block for them.

As you read this book, there is virtually nothing said about exercise until the last section. **EXERCISE IS VERY IMPORTANT** for optimum health—but only when used appropriately. Just be aware that I did not forget it. It will be introduced at the appropriate time.

WHY THIS BOOK?

Unless you live on an island where there is no Internet, television, newspaper, magazine, radio, or any other type of communication, you have undoubtedly heard how obesity has become a serious health problem. Studies suggest that *one in three people is obese* and at least *two-thirds of the population of the United States is significantly overweight* (this is probably a gross underestimate). *Health problems* have accordingly increased, with the leading issues being *cardiovascular disease and diabetes. Nutrition has been given little consideration* of its effects on obesity and development of other health problems including *autoimmune diseases, such as rheumatoid arthritis and various types of cancer.*

For many years, I watched as the obesity problem has continued to grow. **NUMEROUS WORTHLESS** diet programs, supplements, and other schemes aimed at curing obesity continue to be developed **BUT HAVE HAD NO EFFECT**. *This includes the efforts by the medical community.*

Understanding the **TRUE CAUSE OF OBESITY AND KNOWING HOW TO DEAL WITH IT CORRECTLY** are what are lacking in the current fight against obesity. There are bits and pieces of the needed information that are readily available on numerous websites and other information sources. However, **NO ONE** has put this information together in a single source in a practical format **UNTIL NOW**.

How I Got Involved

I currently practice obstetrics and gynecology and have been involved with medicine for more than twenty-four years. However, *I became involved with nutrition and exercise more than forty years ago.* I was in the Air Force, and like many others, I smoked, drank, and was out of shape and overweight. Smoking and being overweight really bothered me to the point that I had to do something about it. During this time, I also realized that my diet was really poor and started researching nutrition. Many nutrition books were studied, including textbooks and those written for the layperson.

I was able to stop smoking after many failed attempts. At the same time, I started a weight lifting exercise program. It didn't take long to realize that eating properly played a huge role in successful weight training. The nutrition information took on a whole new meaning under these circumstances. I started eating more nutritious meals and completely eliminated junk food and as much processed food as possible from my diet.

The search for more nutrition information and better ways to work out did not stop here. I continued to study nutrition and exercise to improve my workouts and nutritional health. Supplements and high-vitamin doses were very much a part of an athlete's diet. After studying enough nutrition information and studying the diets of various athletes, it became apparent that *even extreme athletes frequently ate inappropriate diets.* Some of their diets were comprised of very high-protein intake from good protein sources, such as meat and eggs, but also contained many *unnecessary* supplemental proteins and other nutritional components popular at the time.

Women, in particular, are more concerned about their appearance, especially their weight. As a physician of women's health, I tried to help them learn how to manage their weight in a reasonable fashion without the use of drugs or radical diet plans using the knowledge I had accumulated. As I presented information to them, I could see an immediate response as they realized that the information that they had been hearing and using was wrong. The truth made sense to them, and they started to embrace it immediately.

However, discussions in a clinic setting were not sufficient to adequately educate them on what they needed to know. Also, there was *no additional information anywhere* that could help them establish and maintain a permanent weight-loss and health program. Therefore, I tried to put together brochures and other educational material to help them learn how to eat healthily and achieve their desired weight.

It wasn't long before I realized that this approach was also inadequate. It takes much more information to educate people on how to achieve good health and the weight-loss goals they are seeking in a practical fashion. *The decision was made to write a book that does contain all the knowledge needed to achieve one's weight and, more importantly, health goals and to be able to maintain them for a lifetime.*

People also need to have some basic physiology background with information on how to use this knowledge. Over the years, **I HAVE DISTILLED THIS INFORMATION INTO JUST THE RIGHT AMOUNT** that is necessary to know without generating confusion with too much knowledge. The minute details are purposely left out. If I incorporated a lot of detailed information, this book would be several hundred pages long. This would make it extremely difficult to pick out just the important information. My book would then be just as confusing as the other books and websites addressing dieting, health, and weight loss. It is virtually impossible for anyone to pull together the necessary information to achieve good nutritional health and maintain his or her desired weight (even most well-educated people).

Also, knowing the detailed information will NOT help you learn to eat appropriately. It only adds confusion as you try to control a finely tuned system that is very complex and is already well controlled by its natural programming. Trying to control this finely tuned machine can only result in interference, not improved performance.

THERE ARE NO NEW TRICKS OR NEW WONDER DRUGS TO BE DISCOVERED. You don't need detailed knowledge of human physiology to understand the information you need to achieve your weight and health goals, *just some simple,* **BASIC KOWLEDGE** *that anyone can understand and is* **CONTAINED IN THIS BOOK**.

THINGS YOU NEED TO KNOW

There are a few basic facts that you need to know related to diet, weight loss, and health. Most people I have encountered *do not know or understand* this necessary information. Even if you feel like you know a lot about these topics, I suggest that you read through all this section. There may be some things that you have not considered before. If not, you will, at least, be sure that you know the needed information.

Without this information, you will continue to be tempted to pursue some of the endless barrage of products promising you unrealistic results. *Their advertisements are so good that they sometimes make me feel like I should try their products.* Once you understand the facts that are presented here, you will *know that their products or diet plans are quite ridiculous.* This will save you untold amounts of time and money that you would otherwise waste uselessly in order to achieve your weight goals.

Learning from History

If you look back and take a lesson from history, you *will find some similarities in the pursuit of things too good to be true then and now.* I think that most people have heard of the snake oil salesmen of the Old West. Snake oil was a generic name for many compounds marketed as *miraculous remedies.* Their ingredients were usually secret, unidentified or mischaracterized, and mostly inert or ineffective. A *traveling "doctor"* with *dubious credentials* would come along selling some medicine with boisterous marketing hype often supported by bogus scientific evidence. To enhance sales, an accomplice in the crowd, someone giving a **TESTIMONIAL**, would *"attest"* the value of the product in an effort to provoke buying enthusiasm.

How many times have you heard something like (with many variations) *"Here it is! A new scientific breakthrough! Clinically proven by Dr. X! By taking this pill, you can eat anything you want and still lose weight!"* There are people portrayed in the advertisement who testify or **GIVE A TESTIMONIAL** that they have used that product with great success. They are well-conditioned physically and portray the perfect picture of health. If you read the *fine print*, you will find that it also says, "May require some dieting and exercise to achieve these results." **REALLY?**

SNAKE OIL REMEDIES ARE STILL VERY PREVALENT TODAY. *Nothing has changed except for the method of bringing the advertisements to the public.* People are just as gullible and easily convinced that there is a simple way to cheat Mother Nature as they were in earlier times. They may be more easily deceived today than previously with the belief that science really has discovered these great new wonder drugs. People are convinced that somehow, a simple chemical or diet or exercise program is going to bring them good health and a lean body with minimal effort on their part.

The Plain Facts

If you are overweight, it is because **YOU EAT INAPPROPRIATELY**. You most likely eat a lot of processed food and many high-Calorie, low-nutrition foods (the capitalized form of Calorie is used in nutrition to represent a kcal). Even if you think that you eat fairly nutritiously, you are eating more Calories than you need. Undoubtedly, you are not aware that some of the foods that you consume are not nutritious. To lose that unwanted weight, you have probably tried one or several fad diets and used some sort of medication or supplements with varying amounts of success.

To be lean and healthy, you must know a few things about your body and how to use that knowledge. There is **NO** such thing as taking a pill and then eating anything you want and losing weight. There is **NO** pill that is going to burn your fat away while you do nothing. There is **NO** magic pill! There is **NO** wonder program! There is **NO** such thing as exercising for ten minutes a day three times a week and having a body that looks like the trained athlete demonstrating the program. *There is only you, armed with* **SUFFICIENT KNOWLEDGE** *and* **A LITTLE WILLPOWER** *to use that knowledge that will ultimately allow you to achieve a lean body mass and have good health for the rest of your life.*

Limitations of Knowledge

You need to be aware that every professional (physician, pharmacist, nutritionist, etc.) does not know everything there is to know about his or her field of expertise. This may have been true many decades ago, but the amount of knowledge has increased so much that it is impossible for anyone to be an expert in all areas of his or her specialty. However, several television shows portray physicians as though they are all-knowing experts of medicine.

First of all, your typical practicing professional does not perform the experiments or clinical trials where the information was obtained. It comes from researchers, most of whom are professionals who perform the experiments or clinical trials and then publish their findings. The researchers may also be involved in writing books, where the knowledge in their particular field is summarized. This information is then considered to be the exact truth. Whether it is or not, it is the best information that is available on that subject. It could be close to the truth, or it could be far from reality. It is only the best information that is available at that time.

Topics that physicians are presenting on television shows come from books, the Internet, or other sources. They are just presenting it as though they are the experts. Since they are physicians, they must know everything about medicine, right? Even within their field of expertise, professionals are not going to know all there is to know.

The real experts on any type of scientific information are the people doing the research, not the people using the information, such as your typical pharmacist, nutritionist, practicing physician, or celebrity physician. Additionally, the researcher's expertise is very narrow and limited to the area that he or she is researching. Also, just because someone is researching a subject does *not* mean that he or she knows all there is to know about it or that the information that he or she is obtaining is accurate. Remember the cold-fusion hype from the 1980s? Do you really think that Al Gore invented the Internet?

Medical Science

Considering the great medical advances of our time, **YOU MAY HAVE A HARD TIME BELIEVING THAT MEDICINE CANNOT DO THINGS TO MAKE YOUR BODY FUNCTION BETTER THAN IT IS DESIGNED TO.** Most people have the impression that science knows everything about the human body and that there are drugs that can control every aspect of its physiology and psychology. They are under some kind of delusion that new drugs are being discovered that will modify the body so that it will lose weight while they eat nonnutritious food and somehow be healthy. People assume that chemicals are found that will control their moods or desires (such as drugs to make them want to quit smoking or to no longer crave food), slow their aging, and make them strong, etc., all without having to put out any effort.

MOST MEDICAL PROBLEMS DEVELOP PRIMARILY FROM IMPROPER CARE OF YOUR NUTRITIONAL AND PHYSICAL NEEDS. You continually bombard yourself with poor nutrition in the way of fast food, snack food, carbonated drinks, candy, etc. (not to mention smoking, drinking, and ingesting other harmful chemicals). Treating your body this way results in a shortage of nutritional components. Now it has to deal with excessive amounts of fats, carbohydrates, and other undesirable chemicals or pollutants without the associated nutritional components needed to process these food elements or eliminate the unwanted pollutants.

You further compound the stress in your body by failing to provide adequate physical stimulation that would also help it deal with the excess fats and carbohydrates and undesired pollutants. Over time, this continuous bombardment overwhelms your body's ability to function properly, resulting in high blood pressure, diabetes, cardiovascular disease, many lung diseases (mostly caused by smoking), cancer, and other disease processes.

When your body gets to the point where it is no longer functioning normally, you seek medical care. Most of these problems, especially in the early stages of malfunctioning, *can be corrected by lifestyle changes.* A proper diet will improve nutritional status (nutrition), and exercise will improve cardiovascular and musculoskeletal fitness (functioning). When proper diet and exercise are insufficient or when the patient is unwilling to commit to lifestyle changes, medical intervention may be necessary.

The irony is that even in the early stages of malfunctioning, *physicians prescribe medication* rather than working on ways to promote self-healing with proper nutrition and exercise (mainly due to lack of knowledge about nutrition and exercise on the part of the medical community). Also, since you are going to the doctor, you expect or sometimes demand to be given medication that will correct the problem. Now you are taking medication that, in many cases, has severe side effects, but *you are doing nothing to reverse the process that caused the problem in the first place.*

One such problem is osteoporosis in menopausal women, a condition where the bones thin and weaken, making the person vulnerable to fractures, curvature of the spine, and other related bone problems. Some medications used to treat this condition can cause osteonecrosis (death) of the jawbone and/or severe bone/muscular pain with other side effects. Besides having to deal with the problems from the medication, *you are still pursuing the lifestyle that promotes that medical condition.*

Rather than taking the medication, you should improve your diet, increase calcium and vitamin D intake, and increase weight-bearing exercise. I realize that there are many people who cannot exercise. They just have to do the best that they can with nutrition. However, the number of these people, compared to the number who can exercise, is very small. One point in medicine's favor is that many times, the disease process has progressed beyond your body's ability to self-correct under any circumstances before you seek medical help. However, don't forget the previous discussion on limitations of knowledge.

Natural Medicine and Physical Function

Some companies try to sneak supplements or other products into the available treatment options for various illnesses. These fall under the category of *Natural Medicines*. Most of these products have **LITTLE OR NO SCIENTIFIC EVIDENCE** for their beneficial claims. As an example, *raspberry ketones*, as promoted by a prominent television physician, are claimed to make your fat melt away. However, this has **NOT** been studied in humans and **NOT** demonstrated in animal studies. Similar chemicals demonstrated an increase in lipolysis (breakdown of fat) in laboratory experiments. This led to studies in mice using raspberry ketones that showed a reduction in fat accumulation when they were fed certain high-Calorie diets. This was then extrapolated to this will cause humans to burn their fat stores just by taking this substance. Therefore, there really is **NO EVIDENCE** for the claims made by the producers of this product, and it is **EXTREMELY UNLIKELY** that there is any benefit to be obtained from taking it.

As amazing as some of the pharmaceutical medicines and surgeries are, you still have to realize that there is **NO CHEMICAL, SURGERY, OR OTHER THING THAT IS GOING TO IMPROVE THE NATURAL PHYSICAL OR BIOCHEMICAL FUNCTION OF YOUR BODY** (unless your body was severely deformed at birth). At this point, you are probably thinking of some exceptions to what I have been saying. You remember all the commercials promoting the new wonder drugs that promise great things. Many of them are so convincing that they almost make me believe their claims are true. **IT IS HARD TO LET GO OF THE IDEA THAT MODERN MEDICINE CAN DEVELOP PRODUCTS THAT ACTUALLY MAKE YOUR BODY PERFORM BETTER THAN IT WAS DESIGNED TO OR MAKE IT LOSE WEIGHT WITHOUT ANY EFFORT ON YOUR PART**.

There is a television program where a celebrity physician was promoting red palm oil. What a wonderful discovery this is. This miracle food is a Stop sign for aging promoted to "slow aging, prevent dementia, fight heart disease, and help weight loss." Wow, a product "clinically proven" to help you stay young, have a healthy heart and brain, and lose weight at the same time.

I assure you that I have not misspoken. If such a product really existed, it would be a great scientific breakthrough. Its discovery would appear in many scientific and medical journals, and it would be discussed on every major news program during prime time. The fact is, you only see these products advertised on certain infomercials, and these have become fewer as time has passed.

As you read this book, do not think that I am unaware of the knowledge that medical science has accumulated. Consider how medicine has greatly improved life by interfering with disease processes that were previously very devastating. It is easy to extend these ideas into believing that science can make your body perform in ways that are not possible. All these medical and surgical advances have greatly improved outcomes from previous medications and procedures. Again, none of these advances have changed the way your body functions or improves on the way it functions. Diabetics can take insulin and now some oral medications to help keep their blood sugars normal. They cannot grow a new pancreas to produce the insulin. Even if they could, that would not improve the functional capability of their body but merely replace something that had gone wrong.

Nutrition and Weight Loss

The number of books and websites addressing nutrition and weight loss is overwhelming. A few of these are excellent sources of information; most are not. There is a lot more information than most people want to know and definitely more than you need to know. Although there is a large amount of good information on the Internet, you have to be very careful where it came from. **MOST OF IT IS FROM PROMOTERS OF SOME PRODUCT OR PROGRAM AND IS SKEWED TO FIT THEIR NEEDS.** How do you sort through the enormous amount of information and make sense of it all? For those people who even try, they mostly get confused and frustrated. In the end, they resort to the fad diets or other programs that lay out your diet and exercise programs for you. (If you want a good, unbiased example of this information, go to the website http://Health.gov/DietaryGuidelines/. You will be able to see how confusing even nonbiased information can be.)

The promoters of these supplement and diet programs **DO NOT** try to educate you on how to be healthy and lose weight without using their product. Most people are not educated enough to recognize the ridiculous nature of their proposals. A few people have recognized these fallacies and have tried various ways to counteract the flood of false information.

There are also **NO ORGANIZATIONS WHOSE PURPOSE IS TO DEBUNK ERRONEOUS CLAIMS BY PROMOTERS OF WEIGHT-LOSS PROGRAMS, SUPPLEMENTS, HERBAL REMEDIES, ETC**. If someone has a product or program that is too outlandish or makes too bold of a claim, the Food and Drug Administration (FDA) has occasionally stepped in and stopped them from promoting their product. For example, the B-HCG injections claimed to suppress your appetite were pulled from use because the FDA could not find any evidence that B-HCG actually suppressed the appetite. They did accredit the weight loss from the program to the five-hundred-Calorie diet that you had to maintain while on the injections. This is starving for most people. (Daily Calorie consumption for an average person is around two thousand.)

The FDA requires most food providers, whether the product is processed or fresh, to list the ingredients and caloric content of their products on the labels (if you would like to see the actual requirements, go to the government website referred to above). The labels also contain the breakdown of carbohydrate, fat, and protein percentages and the vitamin and mineral content. In the overall scheme of things, this information is of limited value. It is sometimes handy to use the caloric information to determine if you really want to consume that many Calories.

What you really need to know is how to care for your body so it will function the way it was designed. The irony is that you already know almost everything you need to know to accomplish your goals. The flip side of this is that no matter how much you know, you cannot change what you need to do to be healthy and nutritionally fit. **FORTUNATELY, ALL YOU REALLY NEED TO KNOW ABOUT NUTRITION AND WEIGHT LOSS IS THE INFORMATION PRESENTED IN THIS BOOK.**

Supplements

Supplements are things that you ingest in addition to your regular food. They are considered food products and are **ONLY UNDER THE SAME REGULATION BY THE FDA AS OTHER FOOD PRODUCTS**. Therefore, **ANY CONCOCTION THAT ANYONE CAN DREAM UP CAN BE SOLD AS A SUPPLEMENT.**

There are many supplements and natural medicines advertised to cause you to lose weight or have specific effects on your body. Even if their claims are somewhat correct, **YOU WOULD NOT GET THE EFFECT THAT THEY PROMOTE**. An example is the red raspberry ketone supplement that is advertised to melt your fat away. If it really causes your body to consume fat stores, it would be insignificant. As there is no scientific evidence that the raspberry ketones actually cause fat loss, it is *extremely doubtful* that there is any benefit from its use.

This is a **HUGE INDUSTRY** with a multitude of information being produced to promote their products. However voluminous the information is on nutrition, it is dwarfed by the enormous volume of information by promoters of supplements. **THIS INFORMATION IS USELESS AS IT IS SKEWED TO THE PRODUCTS THEY ARE PROMOTING.** Their information usually has nothing to do with reality, but you don't know that.

You may find yourself saying, "Which one or combination of these supplements do I take?" or "I tried that one, and it didn't work, so maybe I'll try this new one." Over and over, you find yourself trying various supplements without any change in your health or physical status. Most people who supplement shop are trying to lose weight or treat some medical condition and are probably not thinking about nutrition.

It is very difficult to sort out the good from the bad information. So how do you get educated on supplements so you can take the appropriate ones for your needs? Fortunately, just as in nutrition, you don't need to know a lot of information. It is **EXTREMELY** unlikely that you need to take any supplements. Therefore, **IF YOU UNDERSTAND THE INFORMATION IN THIS BOOK, YOU WILL HAVE ALL THE INFORMATION YOU NEED TO KNOW ABOUT SUPPLEMENTS TO ACHIEVE YOUR DESIRED WEIGHT AND BE HEALTHY**.

Diet Plans and Drugs

Diet Plans

When experts analyze the fad diets, they universally arrive at the same conclusion: **THE DIET PROGRAMS ARE ALL FLAWED**. Some claim to provide your body with the "most appropriate nutrients" or "cause changes to your metabolism," thus allowing you to lose weight. Others may want you to assume that they have discovered some secret combination of foods that encourages your body to lose weight. **WHAT REALLY ENCOURAGES YOUR BODY TO LOSE WEIGHT IS EATING FEWER CALORIES THAN YOU NEED,** causing your body to consume some of its fat stores to provide the needed energy for metabolism. *This is exactly what their diet plan provides; but* they usually disguise that fact by directing your attention to something else.

Even if their diet plan is, to some extent, nutritionally balanced, there is an added component. Following it **USUALLY REQUIRES YOU TO REGULARLY CONTRIBUTE FINANCIALLY**. They may offer prepackaged food or require that you purchase some other part of their plan to maintain their diet.

Do you lose weight on these diet plans? Of course you do because they provide **FEWER CALORIES THAN YOU NEED SO THAT YOUR BODY WILL CONSUME SOME OF YOUR FAT** (and unfortunately some of your protein) to make up the difference in the needed Calories. Their plans do **NOT** include teaching you how to maintain a healthy diet independently from them (usually their plan is not a healthy diet). When you can no longer afford their product or reach your desired weight goal, **YOU HAVE NO PLACE TO TURN EXCEPT TO YOUR OLD WAYS.** This is what got you into trouble in the first place. So you end up right back to where you started, except you *are always worse off than before with more weight gain and worse health.*

Many people have studied various cultures and individuals, hoping to discover their secret to longevity and health. From their studies, they have come up with various diets and lifestyles they tout as the **"PERFECT DIET"** or **"PERFECT LIFESTYLE."** The facts on **THE COMMONALITY OF ALL THESE GROUPS OF PEOPLE AND INDIVIDUALS IS THAT THEY EAT A HEALTHIER, BALANCED DIET THAT CAN BE ACHIEVED IN A NUMBER OF WAYS**. This was demonstrated by these people living diverse lifestyles in diverse cultures with similar health and longevity.

Fat Blockers and Absorbers

One of the worst ways to diet is to ingest chemicals that promoters promise will allow you to lose weight without changing your current lifestyle. **I DON'T KNOW HOW MUCH FARTHER FROM THE TRUTH ANYTHING COULD BE.** Some chemicals block digestion of fats such as Alli (also known by other names). Thus, if you eat too many fats, you get diarrhea, which encourages you to avoid fats. This really doesn't work as you avoid the drug to avoid the diarrhea if you wish to ingest fats. Also, if you completely avoid fats, you can easily ingest enough carbohydrates and proteins to allow you to gain weight. In addition, you need fats in your diet to be healthy. So what have you gained by taking this drug?

Appetite Suppressors

The most common diet drugs attempt to suppress your physiological hunger (or the hunger that you feel when you need to eat). The most popular ones in 2015 are Phen375, PhenQ, Hiprolean X-S, Raspberry Ketone Plus, and Garcinia Pure. For a good comparison, read the infomercials on these products and then reread the section titled "Learning from History." *I think you will start to understand the correlation.* These drugs may, in some way, suppress your hunger, *but your weight and nutritional problems are* **NOT FROM FEELING HUNGRY**. The drugs may be more effective if they also cause some nausea, thereby discouraging you from eating, which is the real effect of the drug not the hunger suppression. The most dramatic effect of these drugs is probably from the placebo effect. You expect to not be hungry, so you don't eat.

Cleansing Agents

There are drugs and other concoctions that promise to clear your body of "sludge" or to cleanse your body—again, **AN EMPTY PROMISE**. There are many of these agents/drugs available. Just google *cleansing agents*, and you will overwhelm yourself with information. **YOUR BODY DOES NOT BUILD UP SLUDGE** or, in other ways, store or accumulate debris in your bowels or other organs. Can you imagine how large your organs would get over several years if they did collect debris?

All the folds in the bowel wall increase its surface area, allowing it to absorb nutrients from a smaller volume than would otherwise be required. Sludge or food products **DO NOT** accumulate in these folds. The natural motion of the bowel, combined with components from food, essentially scrapes any material away from the bowel wall.

If any material were to attach to the bowel wall, it would slough off with the lining. This is because the absorptive surface is continuously growing, replacing itself every few days. As the old cells slough off, anything attached to them would no longer be attached to the bowel wall and would also slough and not be able to form sludge. This would be similar to supergluing your fingers together. As the outer dead cell layers that are glued together break loose from the underlying dead cell layers, the glue would lose its hold on the skin, and the fingers would come loose. It may take a day or two for this to happen, but the glue would not have any long-term ability to keep the fingers held together.

TOXINS DO NOT ACCUMULATE IN YOUR BODY. The liver and kidneys are designed to remove them. If you have excessive toxins, it is because you regularly ingest more than your liver and kidneys can clear, or you have liver or kidney dysfunction. Some people claim that sludge in your colon produces toxins that effectively poison your body. *Nobody has* *demonstrated that there is sludge accumulation as explained, and they have not demonstrated that toxins are produced in the colon.* Even if there was sludge buildup and toxin production, the toxins would be cleared by the liver and kidneys. Since there really is no sludge buildup, there is no toxin production. There are bacteria and other organisms that live in your bowel and produce chemicals, but these are not toxic to your body. In fact, most of the organisms are beneficial and help in digestion or making certain nutrients available to your body.

Atherosclerosis

What about atherosclerosis (or hardening of the arteries)? This is a form of sludge buildup, isn't it? Your body is accumulating an excess of cholesterol and storing it in the artery walls, right? Wrong! The body is accumulating cholesterol in the artery walls, but not because there is an excess that just piles up. So far, no one has really determined what causes the malfunction.

The most plausible mechanism is a virally stimulated malfunctioning of your immune system. This causes it to treat certain components of cholesterol as a foreign body in the same way it would a virus or bacteria. Once stimulated, macrophages (large white cells that are part of your immune system) that reside in the blood vessel walls engulf the LDL (the bad) component of cholesterol. Over time, large amounts of these macrophages collect in the vessel walls, forming the plaques. These plaques do not produce toxins and cannot be flushed from your body.

Immune-Mediated Problems

In addition to the atherosclerosis example, there are several diseases that are directly related to the malfunctioning of the immune system. A familiar example is immunologic changes caused by group A strep, a species of bacteria that causes sore throats. Infections from this bacteria result in your body producing antibodies against it, just as it does for every other bacteria. However, these antibodies may mistakenly attack the valves of your heart; this, of course, can result in devastating problems.

Another example is changes in the immune system that cause the body to attack its joints, as in rheumatoid arthritis. In many of these diseases, as in atherosclerosis, viral triggers are suspected as the cause. They stimulate your immune system to produce antibodies that also attack your body. **NUTRITION COULD ALSO BE A CONTRIBUTING FACTOR.** It is rarely, if ever, considered when performing medical studies. *When your body is not provided with the proper types of nutrients in the proper amounts, it could malfunction in a multitude of ways.*

Pollutants

By-products of metabolism and foreign materials within your body are broken down by the liver and excreted in urine or feces. Some are just excreted in the urine. Things that cannot be broken down or excreted are either walled off by fibrous (scar) tissue or engulfed by macrophages (large cells that are part of your immune system). An example of this is tattoos. The ink is engulfed by macrophages. They cannot break down the ink. Therefore, the ink is held within the macrophage until the cell dies. The dye is released when the macrophage is broken down and is again engulfed by another macrophage, and the cycle continues. You may notice that the sharp image originally placed in the skin tends to blur over time. This is one of the reasons this happens. The macrophages slowly move the ink, resulting in deforming the once-crisp lines.

Considering the environment you live in, you are exposed to many pollutants such as automobile exhaust, chemicals used to produce your food, and many other chemicals that come from manufacturing processes or that naturally occur in your area. Great attempts have been made to reduce your exposure to these chemicals, but you still ingest some of them. Let's be realistic; although there are several organizations working to reduce your exposure to these harmful pollutants, *they cannot eliminate your exposure to them.* The only way you can minimize their effects on your body is to ensure that it is functioning at its best and hope that this is sufficient to keep it healthy.

Food Sources

Plants and animals are preprogrammed to function a certain way. Therefore, if they do not get needed nutrients, they cannot perform necessary chemical reactions to grow normally. This is manifest in their appearance and taste. So unless a food source is given appropriate nutrients for it to grow healthily, it will not be as marketable. There may be slight differences in nutritional content of foods grown in different areas and given nutrients from various sources. However, the difference in nutritional content is **NOT SIGNIFICANT ENOUGH** to warrant buying specially produced food. In general, the food available in your local grocery store has all the required nutrients for your body to be healthy.

It is possible for plants and animals to contain molecules that are not part of their normal functioning. Examples are antibiotics and growth hormones. Once the discovery of their presence was made, steps were taken to eliminate them from the products. *Especially with current controls in place by the FDA, the risks associated with these extraneous molecules or possible factors related to the use of farming chemicals or fertilizers are not significant enough to warrant the use of "natural foods."*

You also cannot control the way your body functions; those processes are preprogrammed. Certain chemicals may be ingested that can interfere with natural processes, make them occur at a higher rate, slow down, or stop altogether. Some authors, including some nutritionists, suggest that you should eat some particular food, giving you a certain compound that affects your body in a specific way. Many herbs and supplements are also claimed to have specific beneficial effects.

Although these various compounds may interfere with some function in your body, **THEY ARE UNLIKELY TO BE BENEFICIAL**. Your body is a finely tuned machine. Trying to force it to perform certain functions differently than they are designed to be performed is unlikely to make it function better. *By altering a particular function, you are more likely to throw your body out of balance* than make it perform better overall. In the long term, these compounds **WILL HAVE DETRIMENTAL EFFECTS.** This would be like amplifying the tuba section of a symphony to overpower the rest of the symphony. I doubt that this would make the music more pleasing.

You will be better off by eating a proper, balanced diet that will provide all the necessary nutritional components for your body to function at its best. The only thing that you need to understand is that **ALL THE NUTRITIONAL COMPONENTS REQUIRED FOR GOOD HEALTH ARE CONTAINED IN THE FOOD THAT IS ALREADY AVAILABLE.** You just need to learn how to eat this food appropriately.

Scientific Studies

Producers of dietary aids, supplements, natural medicines, etc., make claims about their products that are supported by "scientific studies" or "clinically proven." These studies are supposed to prove the benefits gained from using their products. *Scientific studies and clinically proven are terms used by these people to entice you into believing that there really is proof that their product works* (you may want to go back and reread the section titled "Learning from History").

First of all, you believe that every scientific study is capable of proving the stated claim. You also believe that the study is performed by a highly trained individual who is the expert in that field; this product was verified through clinical trials performed by Dr. X. Therefore, you believe their results to be accurate and complete. Second, since you don't have enough knowledge in nutrition, you don't question their authority or their ability to conduct or extract meaningful data from the study. You also don't ask to review the information yourself as you would not be able to determine if the study was done correctly, if the data was meaningful, if it had been interpreted correctly, or if they had proven their claim or not (in most cases, the information is probably not available).

Many scientific studies are too time-consuming and have too many variables to extract meaningful data from them. *Nutritional studies are often of this type.* It may require years to get any meaningful data. Also, there may be many uncontrollable factors that bias the study. A group of people randomly selected from a population has very diverse genetic, environmental, and nutritional backgrounds. Some are very fat, some are very lean, some smoke, some eat healthily (most do not), many have genetic diseases that either are isolated to them or run in their families, etc. When you perform a study, you cannot tell which one of the uncontrollable factors may have caused the result you are observing. Many of these studies are performed by examining a population for prevalence of certain health states based on their general diets and environmental exposures. These studies are also fraught with many uncontrollable variables and examiner biases that make these studies of little or no worth.

Obviously, there are some nutritional studies that could demonstrate measurable improvements. For example, if you are studying the effects of vitamin D on rickets, you would definitely see a great improvement as rickets is well-known to be caused by a vitamin D deficiency. If you are looking for the effects of vitamin D on joint aches and pains, you will be very disappointed in obtaining valid data. For one thing, you are looking for a subjective response of improvement from the treatment (how does the participant feel now that he or she is taking the supplement?), not a measurable response such as with rickets.

When studies have no measurable result (such as in joint-ache and virtually all supplement, natural-medicine, and dietary aid studies), *the effect of the treatment is dependent on the participants' interpretation of how they feel.* Therefore, the false positive rate or placebo effect (participants feel like they have experienced a noticeable improvement when they have not been given the treatment) is very high. This false positive rate may be as high as 60 to 70 percent. Studies designed to test the benefit of a certain supplement virtually never demonstrate what the promoter claims, and virtually no one benefits from taking the supplement.

Regulation

The main reason there are so many supplements and other dietary and health products is that there is **MINIMAL REGULATION BY THE FOOD AND DRUG ADMINISTRATION (FDA)**. When you fill a prescription at the pharmacy, you are getting a product that has been through rigorous testing. A panel of professionals evaluates data from the pharmaceutical company to see if it meets certain criteria. If the testing is insufficient to prove their claims with the proper safety profile, further testing is required. The studies are continued until they demonstrate that the drug can provide the desired benefit without harmful side effects or safety concerns. Even with all this scrutiny, medicines have undesirable side effects (just listen to the side effects being given on commercials), and some fail to meet expected therapeutic goals after being prescribed to the general public for a time (just look at all the class-action lawsuits being advertised on television or in magazines).

DIETARY SUPPLEMENTS AND NATURAL MEDICINES ARE NOT SUBJECT TO SCRUTINY LIKE MEDICATIONS. Manufacturers are free to put anything they desire in their products as they are considered food supplements and are only subject to food product regulations. *The same product with the same label could have widely varying amounts of the included ingredients.* Unless their claims are too outlandish or have too many complaints registered against them, they are free to promote their products with almost no limitations.

Health Status

Your body is a complex chemical factory and relies on the availability of certain nutrients to perform as it was designed to. If these nutrients are not available, your body cannot perform to its potential. Take this simple example: If you want to make chocolate milk but you don't have chocolate, can you make chocolate milk? The obvious answer is, of course, no. No one would even consider such a stupid idea, yet you somehow envision your body as being able to perform the impossible by correctly performing billions of chemical reactions without proper ingredients.

Another unfortunate situation is that medicine treats health as an all-or-none phenomenon. No physician would say it in just that way. We all know that there are various levels of health. One extreme is athletes who very meticulously watch their diet, exercise appropriately, and otherwise take care of their bodies to keep them in peak shape. (Not all extreme athletes do this. Some of them cheat or take certain aspects of their diets to the extreme such as very high-protein intake, performance-enhancing drug use, etc.) The other extreme is the couch potato who lies around all day, eats junk food, does little or no exercise, is extremely obese, smokes, drinks, and may do other very unhealthy things to his or her body. Between these two extremes is a spectrum of healthy and unhealthy people.

Also, **A PHYSICAL EXAM AND BLOOD TESTS CANNOT DETERMINE THE HEALTH STATE OF AN INDIVIDUAL.** For example, a physical exam and blood tests are performed on individuals across the spectrum of extreme athletes to couch potatoes. Unless some disease process is occurring in some of these people, there would be no significant differences in their physical exams and lab tests. All the physical findings and lab results would be within limits considered normal for healthy individuals. Therefore, from a medical perspective, if you show signs of disease, you are considered ill. If you don't, you are considered healthy.

Since **YOU CANNOT MEASURE HEALTH,** when medical personnel evaluate a patient, they determine that the patient is either okay (no identifiable signs of disease) or ill (some level of identifiable disease). If the diagnosis of ill is made, the patient may be given medicine to get his or her body functioning appropriately again. In many disease states, this could be necessary as your body may have malfunctioned to the point that it can no longer correct itself without some outside influence such as medicine. **THESE PHYSIOLOGICAL CONDITIONS GENERALLY OCCUR AFTER YEARS OF POOR NUTRITION AND INSUFFICIENT PHYSICAL ACTIVITY.**

I am not naive. I know that there are diseases that are genetically caused or that exposure to environmental substances overwhelms your body's ability to deal with the insult, resulting in a disease state. It's unfortunate that physicians do not as readily recognize predetectable disease states and make corrective action recommendations to avoid the detectable disease states. Some obvious things such as smoking, drinking, cholesterol, and obesity are being monitored, and patients are advised to change their lifestyles to avoid the associated catastrophic consequences and medical costs. **EVEN THESE WELL-RECOGNIZED PROBLEMS ARE INADEQUATELY ADDRESSED BY THE MEDICAL COMMUNITY.** *This is due to the lack of knowledge on how to appropriately and effectively help these individuals achieve significant, lifelong lifestyle changes.*

OTHER THINGS SUCH AS POOR DIET AND LITTLE EXERCISE ARE NOT WELL MONITORED. The recommendations by the medical community for improving diet and exercise demonstrate a lack of understanding of the real issues and the most appropriate approaches to these problems. This is again due to the lack of knowledge about the underlying issues causing obesity and failure at exercising, not to mention nutrition. In fact, this demonstrates a clear misunderstanding in the scientific and nutrition communities in general. They are not discovering the true facts concerning the cause of obesity and poor health because they are distracted by looking in the wrong direction. Therefore, they are **NOT RECOGNIZING THE PROPER APPROACHES TO DIETING AND EXERCISING IN WAYS THAT RESULT IN LONG-TERM SUCCESS IN ACHIEVING GOOD HEALTH AT ONE'S DESIRED WEIGHT.**

IF YOU ARE NOT IN A SOUND NUTRITIONAL AND/OR PHYSICAL STATE, IT'S NOT TOO LATE TO START GETTING YOURSELF BACK TO THE BEST HEALTH YOU ARE CAPABLE OF GETTING. Whether you are a couch potato, alcoholic, drug addict, obese, have many medical problems and are on several medications, have physical limitations or physical deformities either genetically or accidentally, or suffer from many other conditions, *you can still benefit from proper nutrition and exercise within your capability.*

Water Sources

Let's take a look at a label from a bottle of water that came from an artesian well: "Rainfall filters through volcanic rock over hundreds of years, adding vital minerals that give brand X its unique and refreshing taste. The water collects in an ancient artesian aquifer deep within the earth where it is protected from external elements. It's the way nature intended water to be—untouched." Now what these promoters would have you believe is that this particular water source is much better for you than any other water source in the world. They even list the minerals from a "typical" analysis of the water. It was probably only tested once before they started bottling it to make sure it wouldn't poison anyone. From this analysis, they state that it contains silica, calcium, magnesium, bicarbonates and state the pH of the water. This label makes this water sound so good. However, let's look at some facts about water.

First, **ALL GROUNDWATER** (water obtained from wells, whether artesian or drilled) has filtered through soil and rocks to fill the aquifer. In doing so, it loses most of the pollutants from the water and picks up many minerals. Some components are soluble, meaning they dissolve into the water and flow with the water. This is where most of the minerals and other components found in the water come from. Some of the soluble components are not desirable. This includes chemicals from factories, certain pesticides and herbicides, and, in some areas, naturally occurring chemicals. Other components are not soluble and get trapped by the dirt and rocks as water flows through the ground. This filters most undesirable components from the water. Most groundwater contains many more minerals and molecules that are helpful for your body than what this particular label suggests. The mineral list on this water label is very short and would not supply your mineral needs.

The long and short of drinking water is this: *unless you live in an area where the groundwater has been polluted by natural or man-made chemicals, there is no benefit from drinking bottled water.* It may even be less nutritious for you if some of the minerals have been removed to give it a certain flavor or characteristic to enhance sales. Drinking bottled water while in a foreign country (where drinking water purity is not verified and monitored) is probably good to avoid exposure to things that your body is not ready to deal with such as Montezuma's revenge.

IT IS A FACT THAT MOST BOTTLED DRINKING WATER COMES FROM CITY WATER SYSTEMS. It is just filtered with the manufacturer's patented filtration system. Some components could be added to give it a particular taste. Sometimes, the plastic containers come in handy for carrying water or other purposes, but *the effects of the plastic you ingest and how much harm it does to your body have not been fully investigated.* Also, bottled water is controlled by the FDA as a food product, where city water is controlled by the EPA (Environmental Protection Agency). The EPA's requirements are stricter than the FDA's requirements; therefore, *city water's safety is better evaluated and monitored than bottled water*. City water may run through old pipes and is chlorinated, both of which may cause it to have an odd flavor, neither of which is harmful to you. I have a hard time fathoming paying one dollar or more for a bottle of water that someone filled from his or her tap just so you can have "pure, healthy" drinking water.

NUTRITION AND SUPPLEMENTS

When I use the term *nutrition*, I am referring to the components of your food that your body needs to function properly. *The major categories of nutrients include vitamins, minerals, protein, fat, carbohydrates, fiber, and water.* Your body is a complex chemical factory. If it doesn't have the necessary chemicals, it cannot function as it was designed to. Without proper nutrition, it is impossible for you to achieve optimum health and physical strength, overcome or prevent many diseases, have the best mental health, tolerate many stressful situations, etc. **NUTRITION IS THE MOST IMPORTANT KEY TO ALL THE VARIOUS ASPECTS OF YOUR HEALTH**.

The food you eat provides the nutrition for your body. **ALL** the nutritional elements necessary for good health are contained in **UNPROCESSED** food available nearly anywhere in the world. Unfortunately, much of the food supply comes in the form of processed foods in which a lot of the nutrition has been destroyed. Fortunately, unprocessed foods are still in abundant supply and are readily available.

What do I mean by processed food? Anything that you do to a food item that destroys some of its nutritional value is considered processing. Fresh foods have not been through any processing other than washing. Steaming is probably the least amount of processing you can do. Canned food is less nutritious due to the high heat and/or multiple heat cycles used during processing. **VITAMINS** are the nutritional components most sensitive to processing.

At this point, I am going to start looking at specific information concerning supplements, natural medicines, and other substances claimed to help your nutritional state. If there is any sound scientific evidence to support claims made by supplement or natural-medicine suppliers, I will point that out. I am not going to make an extensive search for scientific evidence of their claims as in 99.9999 percent of cases, there is none. In cases where there is scientific evidence, it is of such poor quality as to render it worthless. I will say this, however: *if anyone who promotes any supplement or natural medicine reads this book and takes exception to what I am saying and can prove with **GOOD** scientific evidence that his or her claims are true, I will promote his or her products (I'm not worried).*

Supplements

Using supplements has been promoted for many decades. Most of the first ones attempted to replace some of the nutrition lost in processed food. Currently, there are supplements for virtually anything you can imagine.

Supplements are usually nutritional components such as vitamins, minerals, and proteins. Other supplements are stimulants, dietary aids, energy drinks, and other substances promoted to enhance or alter the functioning of your body. They come in many forms such as tablets, capsules, drinks, bars, and powder. Advertisements say things like "Will give you additional strength," "Be more alert and have more energy," "Lose that unwanted fat," "Will decrease joint pain," "You will get better workouts if you use this supplement." Other supplements claim to cure illnesses, slow aging, increase sexual performance, and improve memory.

They contain such things as caffeine, taurine, glucuronolactone and other amino acids, hormones, neurotransmitters, sugar, vitamins, and many other chemicals. These chemicals are combined in various ways and claim to have beneficial effects. The manufacturers all claim to have research to prove that the chemicals in their concoction will provide the stated benefits. However, **THE REALITY IS, NONE OF THESE PRODUCTS ACTUALLY HAVE ANY HARD-SCIENTIFIC EVIDENCE THAT THEY WORK.** Suppliers are careful to avoid using anything too outlandish so they will not harm anyone. Again, they are under minimal scrutiny by the FDA as they are only considered food supplements, not medications. They take advantage of your naivety and entice you to try their product with the hope that you will cure some illness, be healthier, get stronger, or lose weight faster.

For example, several products promoted to those who exercise claim that you will get a better workout if you take their supplement before, after, or while exercising and that you will burn more energy and lose weight faster. One thing to consider is this: if you can drink anything except a little bit of water during a workout and not throw up, you are not working out hard enough to have any significant physiological effect on your body. These exercise supplements are usually loaded with caffeine and/or sugar to give you an energy boost. *The added protein, sugar, or other components add extra Calories that could be more than you burn during your workout.*

Even for those who work out intensely, **IF YOU EAT PROPERLY, YOU DON'T NEED ANY OF THESE SUPPLEMENTS**. In fact, even if you don't eat properly, you don't need these supplements. **SUPPLEMENTS ARE TOTALLY UNNECESSARY FOR GOOD HEALTH.** This statement is going to raise a lot of controversy, especially with the multibillion-dollar supplement industry. If you have become accustomed to using them to try to enhance various functions, it will be difficult for you to accept the fact that using supplements is not necessary for good health and weight loss. You will have to accept the fact that you **NEED TO USE GOOD FOOD TO OBTAIN YOUR NUTRITION. SAVE YOUR MONEY FOR MORE IMPORTANT THINGS LIKE GOOD FOOD.**

Vitamins

Vitamins and minerals are used as enzymes (or catalysts) in chemical reactions. Enzymes help a chemical reaction proceed more easily. Without getting into a lot of chemistry, let me explain it this way. Suppose you provide food to a group of animals that live in a deep valley where there is no access by vehicle. To feed the animals, you drop bundles of food over a cliff. The bundles of food are delivered by truck, but the truck cannot drive very close to the cliff edge. Therefore, the bundles of food must be carried up a trail where they can be dropped into the valley. The trail is sloped such that on a good day, when you are well rested, you can just barely carry the bundles to the cliff edge yourself. When the bundles of food are brought in on the trucks, the truck driver can stay for a while and help you carry the bundles. The two of you can easily carry the bundles to the cliff and drop them off. When you are finished, the truck driver may stick around for a while or leave right away. If the truck driver is unable to stay or is crippled such that he cannot assist, you must carry all the bundles to the cliff yourself. This results in an accumulation of bundles and could result in starvation of some of the animals in the valley.

The truck driver is like the enzymes that are needed to complete most of the chemical reactions in your body. These enzymes enable the needed chemical reactions to occur at a rate sufficient for proper physiological function. *If the enzymes are not present or do not function appropriately, most of the chemical reactions can still take place—but at a much slower rate, which may not be sufficient for your body's needs.*

Unprocessed foods come with their own truck drivers or enzymes. Processing of food destroys many of the enzymes and other nutritional elements. The environment has many pollutants. These pollutants can also destroy or consume a large portion of the enzymes and nutritional elements. This forces your body to process the food without their help.

For these reasons, many nutritionists have promoted the use of supplemental vitamins and minerals. In the 1970s, the use of megavitamins or large doses of vitamins was promoted. Their claim was, since most of our food is highly processed, the vitamin and mineral components are depleted and should be replaced with supplemental vitamins and minerals. The exceptions to the megavitamin doses are those that have toxicity at high levels. These are mostly fat-soluble ones such as vitamins A, D, and K. Vitamin E may also have toxicity at very high levels. It was claimed that taking large amounts of vitamin C would prevent or cure the common cold.

Time has proven that these megavitamin ideas are false, including vitamin C curing the common cold. Vitamin supplements have proven beneficial in light of the fact that nutritional components such as vitamins and minerals of processed foods are destroyed or lost in processing, and providing them through supplements is beneficial. However, **IT WOULD BE MUCH BETTER TO GET YOUR VITAMINS AND MINERALS FROM UNPROCESSED FOOD.**

Vitamin Requirements

The Food and Nutrition Board of the National Academy of Sciences has established guidelines for the amount of essential vitamins and minerals needed to meet the average daily nutritional needs of most healthy persons. The requirements also vary according to gender and age and are based on a two-thousand-Calorie diet. The amounts are known by the terms *recommended dietary allowance* (RDA) or *adequate intake* (AI).

Another term, *daily value* (DV), which is related to RDA and AI, is used on product labels and vitamin containers. This value indicates how much of a particular vitamin or mineral is contained in a food product or supplement as a percentage of the DV. For example, if a food label shows the percent DV of vitamin A as 10, that item only contains 10 percent of your daily vitamin A requirement.

Your activity level, food intake (including type and amount), body's absorption of vitamins, environmental exposure to toxins, smoking habits, alcohol consumption and physical size all factor in how much of a particular vitamin or mineral you may need on a daily basis. **The DV DOES NOT CONSIDER THESE FACTORS.** Also, your body does not store the vitamins and minerals that are around for only a short time after ingestion. For example, B vitamins are excreted in urine. Within a short time of ingesting vitamin B2, your urine will start to become bright yellow and will remain so for a few hours until its concentration reduces to the point where the urine is its normal color. Some of the fat-soluble vitamins such as vitamins A, D, and E are stored in fatty tissue but still need regular replacement.

Normal amounts of the vitamins and minerals found in your blood have been established, but this doesn't necessarily have anything to do with health. The ranges are established from testing people who are believed to be healthy. Since there is **NO** way to know how healthy any of these people are, **THE RANGES ONLY REPRESENT WHAT IS SEEN IN A PARTICULAR POPULATION.**

The only way to know for sure that you are deficient in a vitamin or mineral is when you start showing signs of disease. People who live in cold winter climates get minimal exposure to sunlight during the winter months. Vitamin D is primarily produced in your skin using ultraviolet energy from sunlight. Therefore, these people need to pay attention to their consumption of vitamin D–containing foods during the winter to avoid becoming deficient. More recently, many people are showing signs of vitamin D shortages in summer and warmer climates due to the excessive use of ultraviolet light-blocking agents and avoiding exposure to sunlight.

THE BEST WAY TO GET NEEDED VITAMINS AND MINERALS IS TO EAT UNPROCESSED FOODS. You will get adequate amounts without supplementation if you eat from all five food groups. Often our food is grown in depleted soil using fertilizer that is much less than optimum. But unprocessed foods still provide the best nutrition available and are not nearly as bad as you might think. Rotation of crops and other farming methods help replenish nutrients depleted by the crops. Also, modern fertilizers do quite well at supplying nutritional components needed by the crops in order for them to grow appropriately and be nutritionally competent.

YOU NEED TO EAT A VARIETY OF FOODS FROM VARIOUS SOURCES AND LOCATIONS TO ENSURE YOU INGEST THE BEST CROSS SECTION OF NUTRITIONALLY COMPETENT FOODS. If any food product is deficient in any nutritional component, that component is likely to be supplied by the same or similar food product being grown in another area. To do this, buy your food from different grocery outlets. They usually do not buy all their food from the same suppliers. Also remember that plants grown in nutrient-deficient soil will not have a healthy appearance and may not taste as good. Just like you, plants must have certain nutrients to be healthy and grow normally. If the food you are eating looks healthy and tastes good, it probably has all the vitamins and minerals usually supplied by that food item.

Organic Foods

You may have noticed that some unprocessed foods are more expensive than processed foods. If you are trying to eat from an organic food store, you will be paying much more for your food. **SINCE THE PESTICIDE AND HERBICIDE CONTENT OF THE NONORGANIC FOOD**, or food produced through commercial farming techniques, **IS NOT SIGNIFICANT COMPARED TO THAT OF ORGANIC OR NATURAL FOOD, THE DIFFERENCE IN PRICE IS NOT WORTH IT.** Also, there is no significant difference in the nutritional quality between organic and commercially produced foods.

The natural foods claim to be grown with natural fertilizers without the use of chemical pesticides and herbicides. Food grown without commercial fertilizers may still be exposed to chemicals that may not be all that good for you. The natural fertilizers such as manure from cows or other animals may be derived from animals fed by crops grown with commercial fertilizers and treated with chemical herbicides and pesticides. If a truly (or as near to *truly* as you can get) chemical, herbicide- and pesticide-free animal or crop is produced (certified organic), it is in such a small quantity to render the volume of food produced insignificant. It is even difficult to grow home gardens in any significant fashion without some element of commercial fertilizer or chemical coming into play.

The reality is that enough food cannot be grown to supply the needs of our population without the use of herbicides, pesticides, and commercial fertilizers. Don't be too nitpicky about this point. *The minimal amount of these chemicals that you ingest is much less harmful to your body than the pollutants from automobiles, factories, smoking (or exposure to smoke), or other harmful chemicals that you are exposed to.*

Free Radicals

Another buzzword or term is *free radical.* I think that this term is also applicable to those promoting diet and supplement programs, but in the context of this book, it refers to molecules that have an unpaired electron. Free radicals really do exist. They come from environmental toxins, chemical reactions, and a variety of other sources, including the normal chemical reactions carried out by your body.

The free radicals interact with other molecules by giving up their unpaired electron or taking one from another molecule. When they take an electron, it oxidizes the other molecule, which could cause it to malfunction. The free radicals are prevented from causing harm when they are neutralized by other molecules called antioxidants.

This is not a new phenomenon or new discovery. Surprise: your body already has a mechanism for dealing with the free radicals utilizing these antioxidants. A variety of chemicals perform this function and are found in many foods. Some vitamins also function as antioxidants. You will hear advertisements promoting various antioxidants including vitamin E, grape juice or wine, and other foods. These various antioxidants are sold as supplements that you don't really need, as they are already found in a proper diet.

Another problem is that these people also advocate using large amounts of the antioxidants resulting in an excess. After all, if a little is good, a lot is better—not necessarily true. Studies show that too much of an antioxidant may be harmful. Once an antioxidant neutralizes a free radical, it can become a free radical. It interacts with another different type of antioxidant that reduces it, but in the process, the other antioxidant becomes a free radical. This process continues with a concert of various antioxidants. They interact with one another, keeping the free radicals reduced, thereby preventing damage to various molecules that could result in tissue or organ damage.

There needs to be a balance of the antioxidants to allow this system to function appropriately. If there is a large excess of a particular antioxidant, it doesn't have enough of the antioxidant that it is supposed to interact with in this concert of antioxidants. *This may cause it to interact with another molecule, causing that molecule to malfunction, which is the process that the antioxidants are trying to prevent.* Therefore, damage occurs to molecules and tissues despite the presence of antioxidants.

This is just another demonstration of using good things in an improper way. **IF YOU EAT GOOD FOOD, FROM ALL FIVE FOOD**

GROUPS, WITHOUT TAKING A VITAMIN SUPPLEMENT, YOU WILL GET PLENTY OF THE VARIOUS ANTIOXIDANTS IN THE PROPER AMOUNTS FOR GOOD HEALTH.

Herbs

This is a good place to discuss herbs. Promoters claim that they supply nutritional components not found in other foods. They make herbs sound like they contain ingredients that will completely change the chemical nature of your body. This herb will make you wise or improve your memory. That herb will improve your immune system. This combination of herbs will cure depression, make you strong, make you more virile, improve your bone health, make your skin younger, or improve your eyesight.

*The chemical or chemicals that can be extracted from the herbs **DO NOT** give the desired effect when given individually or in combinations.* Some interpret this to mean that there is no real effect from the use of the herb. Others interpret this to mean that there is something else in the herb that acts in concert with the detectable chemicals or by itself that is not being detected by the chemical analysis and is providing the desired effect. (I'm sure the tooth fairy left that nickel under my pillow when I was a child.)

FOR THE MOST PART, HERB SUPPLEMENTS ARE MODERN SNAKE OILS. Their manufacturers make bold claims but deliver nothing. Valid studies of herbs usually conclude that "there may be some benefit" from the use of that herb. The key word here is **MAY**. In other words, the investigators could not tell if the desired benefit from taking the herb really existed or not. Remember that right from the beginning, there is at least a 30 and up to 70 percent placebo response during these studies. That is, no treatment was given, but the participant noted improvement of the condition being evaluated. Also, it may take many years to conduct these studies. Virtually none of them (if they are even done) are carried out over a long enough time period to determine a valid outcome.

The end result in nearly all these studies is determined by how the person feels, not a measurable response to the treatment with the herb. For example, if an herb is supposed to give you more energy and make you feel better, how you feel is totally interpreted by you. There is no way to determine how much energy you really gain or how much better you feel. However, if you have high blood pressure, you can be given medications that will lower your blood pressure. It can be measured objectively and is not biased by your interpretation of how you feel when your blood pressure is high. (By the way, many people with high blood pressure state that they can always tell when their blood pressure is high by how they feel. Very well-conducted studies demonstrate that these people cannot reliably tell when their blood pressure is high.)

If there is a valid response to the herbal treatments, it is most likely due to a **DEFICIENCY IN SOME VITAMIN OR MINERAL OR POSSIBLY FROM SOME OTHER DIETARY COMPONENT THAT THE HERB SUPPLIES**. The shortage in the needed nutrient occurs because of an **IMPROPER DIET** on the part of the person taking the herb, not because the person taking the herb could not get the needed nutrient from some other source. So there may be some benefit to a few people who take an appropriate amount of the herb. However, **IT WOULD BE MUCH MORE BENEFICIAL IF THEY JUST LEARNED TO EAT BETTER**.

The bottom line is, chemicals that you ingest do not change the way your body functions. That part is hardwired. You cannot change the chemicals that your body needs to function properly. You can interfere with chemical processes, speed up some functions, slow them down, or stop them altogether. This may seem to be beneficial at first, but as you now know, the alterations become detrimental after a time.

Natural Medicines

Most natural medicines fall into the category of herbs. The only difference is that the manufacturers of natural medicines claim that their product has some effect on your body similar to the effects of pharmaceuticals or prescription drugs. Their claims are not too bold, or the

FDA would make them perform the same studies on their medicines that pharmaceutical companies have to perform on theirs. Similar to herbs, **THESE PRODUCTS FALL SHORT OF PROVIDING THE DESIRED BENEFIT.** For example, menopausal symptoms can be very severe but can be well controlled by the use of estrogen, progesterone, androgen, or a combination of these (usually just estrogen). Many women cannot take these hormones. They may have some medical condition that could be worsened by the use of those hormones, such as women with certain breast cancers. For these women, their menopausal symptoms can be very debilitating.

Some pharmaceutical drugs besides hormones have been used to aid with these symptoms, with a few having predictable benefits. Several herbs, natural medicines, have been advertised to control these symptoms. Some advertise the use of plant estrogens (phytoestrogens) to control menopausal symptoms or to have other hormone effects on the female system. This is appealing to some women, as they don't want some highly processed chemical from a factory when they can use a chemical produced by nature. However, plants *do not* make hormones that behave just like estrogen in humans or other animals. Although the phytoestrogens have similar structures to estrogen, studies show that *they possibly may* have weak estrogen responses in humans. They do provide a substrate or basic chemical that can be modified in a chemical processing facility to behave like estrogens.

If you really want the most natural estrogen, use a hormone that is extracted from a biological organism that produces that hormone. Urine from pregnant horses is one such source. The hormones are totally manufactured by a biological chemical factory, the horse, and are just separated and purified in a chemical processing facility.

The apparent best herbal treatment possibility for menopausal symptoms is the use of black cohosh, also known by many other names. However, the more valid studies can only report, "May be of some benefit." This is again too vague to be useful information. If you try black cohosh and it works, great, but if it doesn't, don't be surprised. **BEWARE OF PROMISES THAT SOUND TOO GOOD TO BE TRUE.** Use your judgment in deciding if you should try a natural medicine, and be honest with yourself whether or not you really benefit from the use of those chemicals. Again, if you do notice a benefit, it is probably because **YOUR DIET IS LACKING THE COMPONENT SUPPLIED BY THE NATURAL MEDICINE**.

Also be aware that many of the herbal and natural medicines can have serious side effects and can interfere with many prescription drugs. If you are on prescription drugs, check with your pharmacist or doctor if you decide to try any herbs or natural medicines.

When a natural medicine seems to be working fine and then quits working, remember that the manufacturers of those products do **NOT** have to consistently include the same ingredients in every batch of product. So if you quit experiencing the desired benefit, a change in ingredients could be the reason, or you may have simply experienced a placebo effect.

IT IS VERY DIFFICULT TO GET RELIABLE INFORMATION ON HERBS AND NATURAL MEDICINES. The information supplied by the manufacturers is too biased and is of little or no use. Also, their research is not readily available to the general public (if it even exists). There are independent organizations that summarize research information from various sources. The problem is that they do not perform the studies themselves. They only have the studies that have been presented from the manufacturers (which are extremely biased) and, in rare cases, from independent studies. Therefore, they cannot make definitive conclusions concerning the efficacy of herbal and natural medicines, but they can give you the best summary of the information that is available.

Most of these are sites run by pharmacists and physicians that do not accept advertising money and, therefore, are not subject to promotion bias. They are accessed by subscription only and may not be readily available to the general public. Unless you can subscribe to one of these sites or know a physician or pharmacist who does, you will not be able to get the best information on these products.

It is best to just forget these products and **WORK ON GETTING THE NUTRITIONAL COMPONENTS FROM YOUR DIET** and not waste your time and money.

ENERGY SOURCES

In general terms, the smallest functional unit of matter is an atom. Atoms are comprised of much smaller particles called protons, neutrons, and electrons. Whenever two or more atoms combine, they form a molecule. Organic molecules are primarily composed of carbon and hydrogen atoms. Oxygen, nitrogen, calcium, and other atoms are also used to make organic molecules. Of course, your body is entirely composed of various types of organic molecules.

The three main types of molecules that your body uses for energy are *carbohydrates*, *proteins*, and *fats*. Don't worry about the structural differences in these molecules. It will not be necessary to understand the differences to use these energy sources wisely. These molecules are used to obtain energy to carry out all cellular functions. These include making specific molecules that your body needs, growing new cells and providing energy to make your muscles contract. Many of the energy molecules are broken down into building blocks used for assembly of other molecules. For example, proteins are comprised of smaller building blocks called amino acids. Proteins you ingest are broken down into the amino acid building blocks and then reassembled into protein molecules that are specific for your body.

It is not important to understand all these cellular functions, but it is helpful to understand a little about energy sources and how your body utilizes them. Keep in mind that the descriptions given here are basic and really all you need to know.

Calories

Calories are a way of measuring the amount of energy obtained from food and other energy sources. One calorie is the amount of energy required to raise one cubic centimeter (cc) of water one degree Celsius. Most people are familiar with the Fahrenheit temperature scale used in the United States. The Celsius scale is just another way to measure temperature change. One degree Celsius is equivalent to 1.8 degrees Fahrenheit.

There are small calories and large Calories. The large Calorie is equal to one thousand small calories or one kilocalorie. In nutrition, the large calorie is used and is referred to as a Calorie. It is capitalized to indicate that it is the large Calorie. I use the capitalized form in this book.

The number of Calories consumed on a daily basis is related to the amount and type of food that is eaten. There is no reference to the nutritional quality of the food, just the amount of energy it contains. **YOUR WEIGHT** is also related to the **NUMBER OF CALORIES CONSUMED** again, **NOT RELATED TO THE NUTRITIONAL QUALITY OF THE FOOD.** If you consume more Calories than needed, you will gain weight. If you consume fewer Calories than needed, you will lose weight. To calculate your daily caloric intake, add up the Calories from the various foods eaten that day.

Carbohydrates

The main energy source for your body comes from carbohydrates. They provide 4 Calories of energy per gram (there are about 28.4 grams in an ounce). These are molecules comprised of chains of simpler molecules called sugar. The sugar molecules are simply connected to one another like links of a chain. As your body processes the carbohydrates, the individual sugar molecules are cleaved from the carbohydrate chains one by one. When the sugar molecules are used for energy, they are broken down in a series of chemical reactions that extract energy from them. This energy is used to drive all the various functions of your body, such as making muscle fibers contract, providing energy to build new molecules and for the growth of new cells. The artificial sweeteners are not carbohydrates. They are a different type of molecule that stimulates your tongue to taste sweet, but they cannot be stored as fat or broken down for energy like sugar; therefore, they have no Calories.

Nearly every type of food has carbohydrates or sugars in some form. Foods that contain higher portions of carbohydrates provide many Calories for a certain volume. Eating a small amount of these foods may provide all the daily energy requirements for your body. Therefore, it is very easy to eat excessive energy that will not be utilized and will be converted into fatty molecules and stored in fat cells. It will be necessary for you to recognize these foods so that you can control your caloric intake better. Foods of this type are flour that is made from cereal grains (which is used to make pasta, bread, cookies, and a host of other products), the meat of a potato (everything inside the skin), the meat of starchy vegetables such as squashes, pumpkins, sweat potatoes, soy, peas, beans, corn, etc. Don't forget that **MANY FOODS CONTAIN A LOT OF PLAIN SUGAR, WHICH IS THE WORST WAY TO CONSUME CARBOHYDRATES**. *The biggest offenders are candy and pop, with other foods such as pastries, cookies and cakes coming in second.*

There are many good books and Internet sites providing the caloric content of food and the proportions of carbohydrates, fats and proteins, so I will not repeat it here. You don't need to know minute details but know generally the carbohydrate content of the various foods so that you can better evaluate your caloric intake. This is not something that you have to master right away and is actually quite easy to do. As you work on improving your diet, you can learn the caloric and carbohydrate content of various foods and learn to eat them in proper amounts. Just remember to consider the possible sugar content of the food item. Labeling on processed and most unprocessed foods has to specify the total amount of carbohydrates and the portion that is from simple sugars.

Metabolism of Carbohydrates

IT IS IMPORTANT TO UNDERSTAND A LITTLE BIT ABOUT THE METABOLISM OF CARBOHYDRATES. When carbohydrates are eaten, blood sugar level rises. The rate of blood sugar rise is dependent on the complexity of the carbohydrate. Sugars have to be cleaved from the ends of the carbohydrate chains. When there are complex carbohydrates (long chains with many sugar molecules per chain), there are fewer ends exposed to cleave sugars from. Therefore, fewer molecules are released at one time. This helps keep the blood sugar lower. When there are very simple carbohydrates (few sugars per chain), there are many ends of the chains exposed, and many sugar molecules are released at a time. This can make the blood sugar rise quickly. Sugar molecules, which are the simplest carbohydrates, are directly absorbed into the bloodstream and will cause the most rapid rise in blood sugar.

To keep the blood sugar within safe limits, *the pancreas produces insulin in response to increasing blood sugar levels. The insulin causes adipose (fat) cells, muscle cells, and the liver to absorb the excess sugar.* This is necessary to keep the blood sugar within normal limits as neural tissue is sensitive to sugar levels and can be damaged by high levels. The excess is also stored for future energy needs. When blood sugar is low, the absence of insulin keeps these tissues from absorbing the sugar. Only tissue that doesn't need insulin to absorb sugar, such as the nervous system, can utilize the remaining glucose.

Once sugar is absorbed into the muscle and adipose tissue, it will not be available later when dietary sugars are not available. The muscles must use their stores for energy and cannot release the sugar back into the bloodstream. The fat cells convert their sugar into fat. When extra energy is needed, the fat is broken down into molecules called aldehydes and ketones. *Muscles can readily use these molecules for energy, but they are not as readily used by neural tissue.*

High blood sugar levels, which result from consumption of simple carbohydrates, *especially sugar,* also cause a **SUGAR HIGH.** This makes you feel euphoric initially with lots of energy. The sugar level drops much faster than the insulin level, resulting in the blood sugar dropping to low normal or below low normal. This results in a feeling of mental sluggishness, nausea, weakness, fatigue, and other feelings resulting from this **INSULIN DOWNER.**

Conversely, complex carbohydrates are slowly broken down. This provides a continuous supply of sugar over a longer period of time. As blood sugar levels do not rise that rapidly, much less insulin is required to keep blood sugar within a safe range. You do not experience the high blood sugar peaks with the corresponding euphoric sugar high or blood sugar lows with the corresponding insulin downer. Therefore, *you avoid this sugar roller-coaster ride.*

When the sugars from a meal are absorbed and the blood sugar starts to drop, insulin production ceases to prevent the blood sugar from going too low. Muscle cells, fat cells, and the liver stop absorbing sugar. As tissues that don't need insulin consume the remaining blood sugar, the level drops lower, signaling a need for more sugar. Remember, muscle cells cannot release stored sugar, and the fat can only be broken down into aldehydes and ketones. So in times of low blood sugar, *the liver releases its stores to maintain a desired level.* Note that during these times, there is no insulin production, so the muscle and fat cells cannot use this sugar. *When the liver depletes its sugar stores, it has the ability to manufacture glucose from protein* to provide the necessary glucose for neural function. The unfortunate thing is, *when your protein intake is inadequate, the protein comes from muscle* and could be from heart muscle or muscle from other organs, not necessarily from skeletal muscle (muscles that make your joints move).

Glycemic Index, Diabetes, and Insulin Resistance

This is a good time to discuss the glycemic index (GI). It is a relatively new term used in nutrition and is used to rank foods according to how rapidly they cause your blood sugar to rise. There is also a corresponding rise in insulin. Those involved with developing this index have made it very scientific, with the goal of helping diabetics maintain better control of their blood sugars. This can also help others who are not diabetic reduce the excessive consumption of simple sugars. By eating foods with a low GI, blood sugar and insulin peaks stay lower. *The lower-GI foods could be associated with fewer health issues caused by high blood sugar and insulin peaks even in nondiabetic people.*

It is fairly obvious which foods will have a high GI. These will be foods that *contain a significant amount of plain sugar.* They are also the foods that you like the best. For example, candy, nondiet pop, cake, cookies, and ice cream are foods that should be readily recognized. Pastas, potatoes, breads, rice, bananas, and many other foods and fruits may not be as readily recognized at first. Although fruits have a significant amount of sugar, they also contain nutritional elements that help your body process the sugar. *All fruits do not have a high GI.* It is not important to know which ones do unless you are diabetic or insulin resistant.

Diabetes (high blood sugar) causes nerve damage. This occurs with all types of diabetes. **MANY PEOPLE HAVE TYPE 2 DIABETES AS A RESULT OF THEIR LIFESTYLE.** It is prevalent in people who are obese and many who eat poor diets. *Nerve damage also likely occurs in any situation where frequent high blood sugar spikes occur, such as the frequent consumption of candy, pop, cookies, pastries, and similar foods.* As nerve damage increases, there is a progressive loss of neural function and often a condition called neuropathy, which causes a burning sensation from the damaged nerves. Persistence of high blood sugar also eventually results in severe organ damage. *You may never test positive for diabetes, but eating large amounts of sugar over many years may result in some organ damage anyway.*

Consuming any **REFINED SUGAR** does **NOT** provide the vitamins and minerals contained in the fruit or vegetable that they were refined from. The body needs these vitamins and minerals to process sugar and perform other functions. Therefore, these sugars are considered **EMPTY CALORIES** and are nutritionally poor energy sources. As you refine your diet, you will eliminate more and more refined sugars. This will help your nutritional state significantly.

HIGH-INSULIN LEVELS are known to cause microvascular damage and will eventually result in organ damage. The insulin levels get particularly high in individuals who have a condition called Insulin Resistance (IR). With IR, your body has to secrete large amounts of insulin to keep your blood sugar normal. This is because *the insulin is not very effective in stimulating fat cells, muscle cells, and the liver to absorb sugar.* Without doing anything to help reduce your body's need to produce excessive insulin, you will sustain severe organ damage after years of high-insulin levels. Many who have IR also develop diabetes that can cause further organ and nerve damage.

High spiking blood sugar and insulin levels occur with frequent excessive sugar intake (frequent consumption of high-GI foods). Excessively high insulin levels occur with undiagnosed IR. The high spiking blood sugar and insulin levels may account for apparent nerve and organ damage in individuals who appear to have normal blood sugar and insulin function. The physical effects of frequent spiking blood sugars and insulin levels have not been studied and never will be due to the complexities of conducting such a study.

The details of the problems caused by diabetes and insulin resistance are beyond the scope of this book. *If you learn to eat healthily,* you will not ingest large amounts of high-GI foods, and you will not suffer or at least significantly reduce the effects of excessive blood glucose and insulin. *If you have several family members with late onset diabetes (diabetes occurring in their thirties or older), it is a good idea to be tested for insulin resistance. If you have it, it is a health issue that you want to start dealing with now (don't be surprised if your physician doesn't know much about IR and how to deal with it).*

Fats

Another energy source comes from fats. The particular structure of these molecules is what defines them as fats, and there are many different forms of them in your body. Fats are used for a wide variety of functions and are used by every cell type. They do not just make your waistline bigger and provide energy when you run out of carbohydrate sources.

A wide variety of foods contain fat, not just meat, eggs, and butter. Many vegetables have a lot of fat as well as nuts and seeds. Margarine, most cooking oil, and a variety of other products are made from vegetable oil, primarily corn oil. *Vegetable oils* differ from *animal fats*, which are *saturated fats,* in that they are *unsaturated fats.* Without getting into a lot of chemistry, let it suffice to say that *your body needs both types of fat, saturated and unsaturated.* For many years, nutritionists and physicians (because of nutritionist recommendations) recommended that you avoid most saturated fats in your diet, supposing that you needed few, if any, of them (mostly to avoid cholesterol or the effects of saturated fats on cholesterol). As more data became available, it was apparent that you need saturated fats in your diet.

Early studies suggested that foods rich in cholesterol (which is also a fat) should be avoided as it contributed to atherosclerosis (hardening of the arteries). From this reasoning, margarines were highly promoted since they are from vegetable fats, which are unsaturated and don't contain cholesterol. A major problem with unsaturated fats used in margarine is that they had to be *hydrogenated* to make them solid at room temperature so that they resemble the consistency of butter.

The process of hydrogenation involves heating the fats to a high temperature under pressure in the presence of hydrogen. *Catalysts*, which are like the enzymes discussed earlier, are needed to help the hydrogenation process happen. Typically nickel or platinum is used as the catalyst. *This process changes bonds in the unsaturated fat into bonds found in saturated fats.* If the process of hydrogenation is carried out to completion, it would convert the unsaturated fat into a saturated fat. This process is only carried out enough to make the vegetable fat solid like butter at room temperature. Therefore, the fats in margarine and many other vegetable oil products are only *partially hydrogenated.* This makes them partially saturated and partially unsaturated. It also eliminates some of the benefits, if there really are any, from eating a purely unsaturated fat.

More recent evidence, now several years old, demonstrated that there *could be harmful effects from eating the partially hydrogenated fats.* They may contribute to atherosclerosis (hardening of the arteries), which is ironically what they were promoted to prevent. Other concerns are for development of cancer, degenerative diseases, increased inflammation, accelerated aging, interference with the immune system, and healing. Evidence now also supports the use of **BUTTER AS A HEALTHY FAT.** Besides providing saturated fats*, it contains many nutrients and vitamins* *not found in vegetable fats.* As you may have noticed, **THESE FACTS ARE NOT HIGHLY PUBLICIZED**.

Fats are a necessary part of your diet and need to be consumed in appropriate amounts to ensure proper nutrition. As an energy source, fats have more than twice the Calories per gram as carbohydrates and proteins *(9 Cal/gm vs. 4 Cal/gm)*. Therefore, avoiding fatty foods or unnecessarily fatty foods such as french fries and breaded foods that are fried in oil can significantly reduce your caloric intake as well as improve your nutritional fitness. *Fast-food restaurants generally use partially hydrogenated vegetable fats to do their deep-fat frying.* This provides not only more Calories from the fat but also partially hydrogenated vegetable fats, which you now know are not good for you.

Eating a well-balanced diet with vegetables and a moderate amount of meat will provide adequate fat for nutritional needs but keep Calories to a minimum. Eating less fatty meat will also help. Reduce (not eliminate) your intake of meat from animals that marble the fat through the meat such as beef and other hoofed animals. This does not mean that you should avoid beef but that you should eat it in proper proportion to the other foods that you eat. Fish and fowl carry their fat on the outside of the meat. Therefore, it can be easily removed to reduce your fat intake.

Cholesterol

Since cholesterol gets so much press, it needs to be better understood. Cholesterol is a *group of fats* that are used in most cells of your body. They are used in the cell walls, in other structural components, and for other purposes. They are the precursor molecule for all the steroid hormones, including testosterone, estrogen, progesterone, and several other hormones. They are important molecules your body cannot do without. *They are so important that if you don't have enough in your diet, your body will manufacture them.* The levels are *regulated* so that your body does not accumulate an excess. If you eat enough cholesterol, your body will not manufacture it. Otherwise, it will manufacture what it needs.

As with any other part of a biological system, if something can go wrong, it will. Certain individuals will manufacture cholesterol, whether they eat it or not. Others may not absorb cholesterol appropriately. Some of these people may benefit from reducing cholesterol in their diets. They may also require medication to help keep their cholesterol within reasonable limits.

Low-density lipoproteins (LDL), which are a component of cholesterol, are associated with atherosclerosis (hardening of the arteries). Current recommendations suggest that keeping LDL to a lower level helps reduce the rate of plaque buildup. This plaque or atherosclerosis is the main issue concerning cholesterol. It is a big issue because as atherosclerotic plaque builds up, there is a major concern for cardiovascular health.

More recent research has discovered that the type and amount of fat you eat appear to have as much influence on cholesterol levels as the amount of cholesterol eaten. Also, the levels of the various types of cholesterol that were previously used as target healthy levels are not as appropriate as believed. Newer evidence is now finding that carbohydrate intake, including type and amount, has a large influence on cholesterol levels. **FOR REASONS SUCH AS THESE, IT IS BEST TO EAT A WELL-BALANCED DIET AND NOT PAY ATTENTION TO ALL THE HYPE THAT IS CONSTANTLY BEING PROMOTED AND CHANGES FREQUENTLY AS NEW INFORMATION IS OBTAINED.**

Your **LIFESTYLE CAN HAVE A PROFOUND EFFECT ON CHOLESTEROL METABOLISM** even when the regulatory mechanisms function appropriately. An important part of cholesterol metabolism is *burning the excess for muscle fuel.* Unless someone has regulatory problems with cholesterol, as mentioned previously, exercising will help keep cholesterol within normal levels.

The detailed metabolism of cholesterol and its various components are complex and well beyond the scope of this book. Let it suffice to know that cholesterol is an important fat that your body cannot do without. **WHEN YOU EAT AND EXERCISE APPROPRIATELY, YOUR BODY WILL TAKE CARE OF THE CHOLESTEROL.**

Proteins

Proteins probably get more press than the other energy sources because they are involved in so many functions. *Every cell has many proteins* used in a wide variety of ways. These range from cell identification to transport of molecules across cell membranes and many other cellular processes. Proteins are an *important part of your immune system.* Proteins, more so than fats and carbohydrates, are *used in virtually every functioning aspect of your body.* Many people think that you have to eat large quantities of protein to make your muscles big. Proteins have 4 Cal/gm, the same as carbohydrates.

There are *twenty amino acids* used in manufacturing all the different proteins. Your body can manufacture eleven of these amino acids (nonessential) but must obtain nine of them from your diet (essential). You could consider these amino acids like building blocks or pieces of a Lego set. Used in various combinations, millions of differently shaped molecules can be manufactured. *Your body will not be able to produce certain proteins if your diet is deficient in any one of the essential amino acids.* This could cause significant malfunctioning of your body, depending on the proteins that cannot be made. (Newer information now suggests that there are at least twenty-two amino acids and as many as two hundred. However, it is still believed that there are only nine essential ones.)

This is why it is so important to maintain an appropriate protein intake. *People who eat a very select diet may have a difficult time consuming a balance of amino acids.* For example, soy contains all nine of the essential amino acids but has disproportionally small amounts of methionine. It is also deficient in cystine, but this is a nonessential amino acid that your body can produce.

Vegetables also contain larger amounts of fats and carbohydrates compared to proteins than other food sources, depending on the vegetable, of course. Therefore, *if you do not eat from food sources with higher proportions of protein per volume of food, you must meticulously control your diet to ensure adequate amounts of the essential amino acids while not overconsuming carbohydrates and fats.* Grains also contain significant amounts of carbohydrates and fats in proportion to proteins. This can contribute to excessive caloric intake when trying to balance proteins, carbohydrates, and fats.

As an energy source, *proteins are very versatile.* They can be broken down by the liver and used to make glucose when there is a shortage of carbohydrate energy sources. Your body's need for protein is so important that *during times of starvation (or other protein-deficient states such as poor diet and high fat and carbohydrate diets), your body will break down muscle tissue to obtain the amino acids needed to carry out essential body functions.* The unfortunate thing is that your body is not particular where the protein comes from. It just randomly catabolizes (like cannibalize, except the body is eating itself) from its protein stores (your muscles)—cardiac (muscle in the heart), skeletal (muscle that makes your joints move), or smooth (muscle that helps organs function, including bowel and blood vessels). *Without the ability to catabolize proteins, your body would fail during times of starvation.*

Diets

Diets are comprised of the things you eat. They may contain an excess or have a deficiency of any or all the energy sources. They may have a balance of energy sources but lack nutritional elements necessary for good health, especially if you eat a lot of processed foods.

It is impossible to eat a perfect diet, as perfect food sources are not available. Many people promote eating natural foods or health foods or organic foods. They claim that these foods have not been exposed to pesticides or herbicides or other potentially harmful chemicals such as commercial fertilizers. But where do they get their fertilizers? And how do they keep insects and other pests from damaging or destroying their crops? For the most part, these terms are just buzzwords to make you think that they are healthier. In some instances, this may be true to a small degree, but it is essentially insignificant. *What you need to be thinking about is learning how to make the things you eat the most nutritious while balancing the energy sources for your body's needs.*

FOOD PYRAMIDS

Food may be divided into groups of nutritional commonality. There are **FIVE MAJOR FOOD GROUPS**. These are cereal grains, vegetables, fruits, meat or proteins, and dairy. **YOU NEED TO EAT UNPROCESSED OR MINIMALLY PROCESSED FOOD** from each one of these groups on a daily basis to ensure that you get all the nutritional elements necessary to be as healthy as possible.

Fruit is the part of flowering plants that contains the seeds. Therefore, tomatoes, squashes, eggplants, cucumbers, cereal grains, nuts, and many other food items are technically fruits. Vegetables are from either the plant's roots (carrots and potatoes), stems (ginger and celery), leaves (lettuce and spinach), or flower buds (broccoli and cauliflower). In general, if the food item comes from a plant and has seeds (except for things genetically cultivated to not have seeds such as seedless grapes), it is a fruit; otherwise, it is a vegetable. These facts can become confusing if you try to make it technical.

Since there is so much ambiguity between some fruits and vegetables, I will use the culinary approach to separating them—that is, how you typically see fruits and vegetables separated in a grocery store. If there are any important distinctions to be made, I will point them out.

Various authors have placed these food groups into food pyramids to help you visualize proportionally how much to eat from each group on a daily basis. The foods eaten in the largest volume are placed on the bottom. Foods at the top should, therefore, be eaten in the smallest quantities. Note that if you search for *food pyramid* on the Internet, you will literally find hundreds of variations. Do not let yourself be confused by all this information. Appendix 1 is an example of a classical food pyramid representing the five major food groups. *This breakdown provides a reasonable relationship of the food groups without making it too complex.*

Appendix 2 is an example of a more recent idea on classical pyramids putting vegetables at the bottom. This represents the suggestion that you should eat a larger volume of low-Calorie vegetables. This is not a bad idea for our current society. You tend to be less active and require fewer Calories in the form of carbohydrates and fats. However, you do need an increase in nutritional components contained in the low-Calorie, high-fiber vegetables, especially with the amount of processed foods that you eat. Appendix 3 is a vegetarian pyramid. Notice that cereal grains have been moved back to the bottom. In general, vegetarians need the protein component from grains and beans.

If you look at a variety of food pyramids, you will notice that many people separate several foods from their common category or subdivide these five categories. For example, green beans are considered vegetables, but the mature bean is more similar to cereal grains and is contained in the meat/protein group by some. Nuts, seeds, and oils are sometimes put into separate groups. Some authors put butter in its own group. Because the major nutritional components in dairy come from the cream, if you don't drink a sufficient amount of whole milk, you need to eat butter in order to get them. You will also see foods grouped under high glycemic index. This includes fast foods and those containing lots of added sugar. Since you are trying to eat healthily, it is best to leave these foods out of your groups. *No matter how you slice and dice it, you need to learn to eat appropriately from the five major food groups and leave the highly processed and sugar-containing foods at the store.*

As I discuss food pyramids, I am not going to fully address the nutritional components of all the different foods. I will give you enough information to help you discern categories of food and how to proportion them. This will be adequate, except for looking up some caloric information. There are plenty of good books and websites providing detailed information on caloric and nutritional components of all foods. This can be overwhelming if you are not careful. If you want to look up information, just look for what you need at that time and ignore the rest. *Don't be deceived or distracted by all the associated diet plans and other information that you find in those books or websites.* Also, **KNOWING**

THE CALORIC AND NUTRITIONAL INFORMATION IN DETAIL WILL NOT HELP YOU WITH YOUR DIET. *Too much information just causes more confusion and causes you to go off on tangents that will take you away from the real issue of just learning to eat proper amounts of good food.*

The grain, vegetable, fruit, protein, and dairy groupings make the most sense (see Appendix 1 and 2). They put foods into the best commonality groups without making it too complex. Many will say that this is not good enough. But let's get real. *The more you chop up these groups and the more complex you make it, the more confusing it becomes and the more difficulty you will have trying to make your diet work for you.*

Vegetables

In general, the vegetables with the highest fiber content have the greatest amount of nutritional components and fewer Calories. Those with the least amount of fiber have fewer nutritional components and more Calories. Other vegetables are between these two extremes. *As a general guide, the less pulpy the vegetable is, the more fiber it contains, along with more nutritional components and fewer Calories.* Pulp is the soft center part of certain vegetables such as in corn, peas, potatoes, and squashes. Just remember that there can be a fairly large difference in Calories between similar vegetables such as peas and corn. Just look up the ones that you are not sure about.

For example, lettuce, cabbage, spinach, carrot, celery, broccoli, cauliflower, green bean, brussels sprout, radish, and many similar vegetables have few Calories per volume but do provide a lot of nutritional components (vitamins and minerals) and indigestible components (fiber). Therefore, you can eat as many of these vegetables as you can tolerate.

One group of vegetables has a softer, pulpier center. This consists of things like corn, peas, and beans. These have a higher content of carbohydrate, protein, and fat but still provide many nutritional components and fiber. Many of these vegetables have a large amount of Calories per volume such as corn and beans. Although they are a nutritious group, you may have to eat from them very judiciously to avoid overeating.

Another group includes potatoes, sweet potatoes, yams, squashes, pumpkins, and similar vegetables. They all have a carbohydrate-rich, meaty (pulpy) center, with varying amounts of skin or peel. In order to take advantage of the nutrition provided by these vegetables, you need to eat all the vegetables (don't throw out the skin or pulpy center). These types of vegetables may also provide more Calories than you need and may need to be consumed in small quantities or not at all.

The five-group food pyramids I am presenting do not divide the various vegetables by their fiber, carbohydrate, or caloric content. Doing so just makes the pyramids very complex and confusing. Therefore, *you need to learn which vegetables can be eaten freely and which ones are going to provide extra Calories with less nutrition.* **THIS IS VERY EASY TO DO, AND I HAVE ALREADY POINTED OUT SEVERAL EXAMPLES.** For the vegetables you are not sure about, look up the Calories using a reference book or look them up on the Internet. Some search engines such as Google will display all the information you will need by just typing something simple like *calories in peas*. Be careful when you use websites that you don't get distracted by other information that may be there.

Note that there is value in eating from a wider variety of vegetables even if some of them are higher Calorie. *Not all vegetables contain the same nutritional components.* Also, some may contain varying amounts of the nutritional components they are capable of providing due to variations in the soil, fertilizers, and other growing factors. *Since all vegetables are not grown in the same location, eating from a wider variety will ensure that you will get the best possible complement of nutrients provided by those vegetables.* **THIS FACTOR ALSO APPLIES TO ALL THE OTHER FOOD GROUPS.**

Cereal Grains

Cereal grains are probably the most widely used group. It is primarily comprised of wheat, barley, oats, rye, and rice. There are several less-known members of this group such as amaranth, millet, quinoa, sorghum, and teff. Corn is also dried and ground into flour to use in making bread or similar products. Even beans can be ground into flour. The one thing all these grains have in common is a *good balance of carbohydrates, proteins, fats vitamins and minerals.* Each type of grain has its own unique combination of these elements.

On older food pyramids and many newer ones, grains are still on the bottom of the pyramid. When you think of all the products that use flour, you can see that *wheat is used in almost everything.* All the different breads, noodles, cakes, cookies, crackers, etc., use wheat or some cereal grain as a major ingredient. Even foods that would not appear to use flour such as sushi, chocolate, and hot dogs usually contain some wheat products.

One of the characteristics of this group is that some of them contain *gluten.* This is a big issue for those with an allergy to it. The highest concentration of gluten is found in wheat, barley, and rye. Sometimes, it is removed from these grains to an accepted level of twenty parts per million (twenty ppm) and used in gluten-free foods.

Soy is noted for having high-protein content, which is true. However, *it is deficient in one of the essential amino acids, methionine.* To achieve a proportional methionine intake, more protein is ingested than needed, along with the associated carbohydrates and fats. This results in a higher-than-needed caloric intake, making it less than ideal as a protein source. However, it continues to be promoted as being equivalent to meat or is considered even better by some people. Just try some tofu meat or tofu bacon, and come to your own conclusion. Another thing to consider is, if tofu is so good by itself, why do people try to make it look and taste like meat products?

Some vegetarians might argue that meat consumers would get as many excess Calories by eating meat that is rich in fat. This may be true, except you can eat meat that has less fat content, such as chicken or fish, or eat leaner cuts of red meat. The main thing to consider, whether you consider yourself a carnivore, omnivore, or vegetarian, is that *you need to learn to eat the proper amount of protein without getting an excess amount of Calories.* (Humans are omnivores.)

Although cereal grains are a basic nutritional food, they do contain a significant amount of Calories. Therefore, several authors of pyramid charts now put them higher on the pyramid, indicating that they should be eaten in smaller quantities than vegetables (see Appendix 2).

Remember that some vegetables also have a significant number of Calories and could be moved higher on the food pyramid. Maybe a pyramid should be built with the highest-caloric foods on the top and the lowest-caloric foods on the bottom. However sensible this may sound, the old five-group pyramid reminds us that eating from the different groups according to the pyramid helps keep our caloric and nutritional components in a reasonable balance. *When eating cereal grains, remember to eat more coarsely ground grains and whole grains.* White flour acts similarly to sugar and can make your blood sugar rise very quickly.

Fruits

Fruits are a very nutritious food group. They contain many vitamins, minerals, fibers, and antioxidants (which has become a popular buzzword to sell products). I say *buzzword* because fruits have always provided these antioxidants. Now they are overemphasized and extracted to sell as supplements. Don't get caught up in this hype. Just eating the fruit provides ample antioxidants. Other foods also contain them, so don't worry about trying to get enough. Just eating a well-balanced diet will provide plenty of antioxidants.

Fruits also contain relatively large amounts of fructose. Their higher-sugar content is one of the things that make these food items classified as fruits and not vegetables. Fructose is slightly different from other sugars such as glucose and sucrose and is processed differently by your body. However, fruits contain the vitamins and minerals necessary to process it. Unless you are eating large amounts of refined fructose, you do not need to worry about how it is used by your body. Fructose is a component of soft drinks, candies, cookies, and many other foods, but any refined sugar contained in processed food is not the way that you should consume carbohydrates.

So in general, *avoid refined sugars, **DO NOT** avoid fruits, and eat a* *wide variety of them.* You can use fruits to help adjust your peak-caloric intake, but do not avoid them to keep your Calories down. Go after the higher-caloric foods produced from flour, soy, potato, and rice first. You need to **ALWAYS** consume some fruits in a wide variety to maximize your nutritional health.

Protein

Protein is contained in many food types such as meat, eggs, milk, cereal grains, and some vegetables. *Meat is mainly comprised of proteins and provides the highest percentage of protein per volume.* It is divided into categories: cloven-hoofed animals—cattle, sheep, and pigs; poultry—chicken and turkey; fish—many varieties; and seafood—mainly shellfish such as crabs, lobsters, shrimps, oysters, mussels, and clams. *Meat contains amino acids in proportion to your basic needs.* Proteins from cloven-hoofed animals generally have fat marbled (layered) throughout the muscle, which results in higher-caloric content per volume than other protein sources. Buffalo is an exception to this rule as its fat is not marbled throughout the muscle but is contained on the outside. Fish and poultry also have their fat layered outside of the meat, making it easy to remove.

Years ago, it was thought by many nutritionists that saturated fats found in animal protein were not needed in our diets. Therefore, they promoted unsaturated vegetable fats (even the partially hydrogenated ones that you now know are not good for you). Research since then demonstrates that you really do *need some saturated fats from animals.* Therefore, if you just eat meat in proper proportion to the other food groups and in proper relation to your caloric needs, you will have what your body needs.

One thing to consider about red meat is the *iron* content. Red meat is red because the muscle cells have myoglobin molecules that contain iron. *This is a source of easily absorbed iron in a form that is most usable for your body.* Leafy green vegetables also contain iron, but in amounts that require large portions to get adequate nutritional iron. For example, a 3-ounce (85 gm) piece of beef would have about 2.2 mg of iron. It would require 8.25 ounces (234 gm or 3 cups) of spinach to get equivalent iron.

Most oral iron supplements are not absorbed very well, and even taking large amounts of them will not increase their absorption. *Getting nutrition directly from your diet is far better than trying to supplement it.* Like the other food groups, you have to learn to eat meat in proportion to your needs. Again, if you are a vegetarian, you can get enough protein and iron, but you have to be very aggressive in making sure you eat proper amounts of the appropriate vegetables (or nonmeat foods).

Before leaving the protein group, note that eggs are usually included in this group. Eggs are very high in protein but are also high in fat and other nutritional components. *If there is one food item that comes closest to being perfect, it is an egg.* It is the only food that contains all the nutritional components, carbohydrates, fats, and proteins to grow an entire organism, a chicken. Some might counter by saying that these are proper amounts for a chicken, but not for a human. They would also state that eggs contain a lot of cholesterol and are, therefore, not good for you. These people overlook two important facts. There is no single perfect food for humans, and it's not the dietary cholesterol that is the problem. *If you had to pick one food that provides the largest variety of nutritional components in the largest amounts that provides good nutrition for humans, that would be eggs (but you have to eat the yolk too).*

The *cholesterol* component of eggs is *not a factor* for virtually anyone, especially someone who is nutritionally and physically fit. (You may want to review the other sections addressing cholesterol.) It may add a bit of complexity for someone who is fat and has cardiovascular disease, but virtually everything does for that person. The main idea here is to not become that person. Also, *vegetarians would have a much more difficult time with nutrition if it were not for eggs.*

Fatty Acids

One of the nutritional components of eggs is omega-3 fatty acid *(which is found in the yolk).* However, chickens producing eggs that are only allowed to eat some commercial chicken foods are lacking something they need to produce fatty acids. If their feed is supplemented with kelp or if they are allowed to feed in an open barnyard, their eggs contain the omega-3 fatty acid. They can also be fed seeds containing omega-3 fatty acid, which helps them provide it in their eggs.

Although you may not get the omega-3 fatty acid from eggs, there are other sources such as fish, seafood, flaxseed, and many others. Therefore, even if you know nothing about nutrition but *heed my advice and eat from a wide variety of foods, you will still get the omega-3 and the other fatty acids.*

I only point this out because some nutritional components such as omega-3 fatty acid are receiving so much press. This happens every time someone thinks that he or she has found a new breakthrough in how some nutritional component is used by your body. **THIS NEW DISCOVERY BECOMES THE FOCUS OF A LOT OF NEW PRODUCTS AND ADVERTISING**. If you eat an extremely poor diet (and many people do), this may be a factor. Those who eat a reasonable diet, even if it is not the best diet, usually get enough of these nutritional components to be reasonably healthy. Again, *the key is to eat from a wide variety of unprocessed food from all the groups.*

Dairy

Some authors break dairy up into product components such as milk, cheese, cottage cheese, yogurt, etc., and put these at different levels on the pyramid. Others suggest using the low-fat versions (to reduce caloric intake, not optimize nutrition). However you break it up, **THE MAIN COMPONENTS ARE CALCIUM OBTAINED FROM THE MILK COMPONENT AND NUTRITION OBTAINED FROM THE CREAM COMPONENT**. The milk component does contain milk sugar (lactose) and some protein. However, milk is not your main source for carbohydrates and proteins. It does contribute to your total caloric intake, so you have to consider that when you are looking for Calories to eliminate. Try to find other less nutritionally significant foods to eliminate before eliminating or reducing your dairy products.

Since a large number of people don't drink milk, some authors put butter into its own food group. This emphasizes that if you don't eat dairy products that utilize the butterfat component, you miss the major nutritional benefits from the dairy group. I would have to agree with these authors. Consider dairy in two parts: **MILK** (and products made from the milk such as yogurt, cottage cheese, and cheese), which provides calcium and some protein and sugar (lactose), and **BUTTER** (*or cream*), which provides the nutritional component and some fats. Also, don't forget that pasteurizing and removing cream from the milk destroys a large portion of its nutritional components.

HOW MUCH DO YOU EAT?

As you start to work on your diet, *use the food pyramid only as a guide to the relative amount that you should eat from the various food groups*—in other words, how many vegetables you should eat compared to the amount of meat, fruits, etc. On the food pyramids in Appendix 1–3, I have listed a range of servings for each food group that is typically recommended. For example, in the cereal-grains group in Appendix 1, it is suggested to eat 4–8 servings on a daily basis. A *serving* could be a cup, a quarter pound, a slice of bread, a single item such as a carrot or potato, or other unit of measure.

In the big scheme of things, *the actual quantity of a serving is really irrelevant.* You have probably already established an idea of how much you like to eat of a particular food item during a meal. *Use this amount as **YOUR** particular serving.* As you learn to eat better nutritionally and appropriately, you will adjust this amount to fit your needs. Just remember to **EAT FROM THE VARIOUS FOOD GROUPS IN THE PROPORTIONS SUGGESTED BY THE PYRAMIDS.**

In June of 2011, the United States Department of Agriculture (USDA) replaced the food pyramids with a new plan for determining portion size called MyPlate. They thought the pyramids were too confusing in determining how much to eat from each group. However, as the portion size is really immaterial, MyPlate is just as confusing as the pyramids. The food pyramids merely suggest how to proportion the different food types (i.e., vegetables need to be eaten in larger quantities than cereal grains, which are eaten in larger quantities than fruits, etc.) as depicted on the pyramids (see Appendix 2). Since the pyramids depict this very clearly, I will continue to refer to them. If you would like more information on

MyPlate, go to the USDA's website: http://ChooseMyPlate.gov.

DO NOT *measure your food or count Calories very closely***.** Let me say that one more time: **DO NOT, UNDER ANY CIRCUMSTANCE, MEASURE YOUR FOOD OR COUNT YOUR CALORIES VERY CLOSELY.** I know that this contradicts everything you have heard, but it just adds stress to learning to eat appropriately and does not help you lose weight. Your body will tell you how you are doing on Calories as you monitor your weight. *Nutritional status is something that cannot be measured.* Therefore, you just have to try to eat the best you can from all the various food groups. Obviously, if you get scurvy, you are not getting enough vitamin C. However, if you eat appropriately from all five of the food groups, as I am recommending, you will not have to worry about being nutritionally deficient.

You will notice that I mention several times that you need to eat sufficiently or appropriately for your needs. What does this mean? **IF YOU ARE EATING APPROPRIATELY FOR YOUR NEEDS, YOUR WEIGHT WILL REMAIN STABLE AT ITS CURRENT VALUE.** It does not matter whether you eat good, nutritious food or junk food. You are merely supplying the number of Calories your body needs to maintain your current weight. It has nothing to do with your **NUTRITIONAL HEALTH**, which is strictly determined by the **QUALITY** of the food you eat. Remember, true health is not measurable.

Vegetables

Vegetables are a diverse group nutritionally and in their caloric content. Therefore, if you are not careful, it is very easy to eat too many Calories. For example, you love corn, peas, potatoes, and squashes and eat them several times a week. If you are trying to lose weight, you need to reduce your consumption of these and similar vegetables. Wean yourself so that you only eat each one of these vegetables one or two times a week at most with small portions. *Get to know the higher-caloric vegetables, and eat them more sparingly* (don't ignore them).

High-fiber/lower-caloric vegetables such as lettuce, cabbage, brussels sprout, cauliflower, broccoli, carrot, celery, radish, tomato, and many others should be worked into your diet. It is very easy to get the suggested three to six servings by combining some of these into a salad or just eating them individually. These vegetables *may be eaten in liberal quantities* (if you are not adding a high-Calorie dressing or eating them in a high-Calorie sauce). Remember that **THESE VEGETABLES ARE GOING TO PROVIDE A MAJOR PORTION OF YOUR NUTRITIONAL ELEMENTS**. There are enough different high-fiber/low-Calorie vegetables that you may only have to eat each one once or twice a week. If you don't have a big enough selection to do this, just eat from the widest variety that you can. You will probably find that it will take some experimenting to expand your variety, but this will be a fun project as you work on changing your diet.

Cereal Grains

Cereal grains are difficult to avoid as they are found in virtually every commercially produced food. Therefore, it is very easy to consume an abundance of Calories from them. For example, you may like to eat pastas, cookies, crackers, etc. These can make up your entire four to eight servings from the grains group. However, as these items are low-nutrition, high-Calorie foods, they should be **WEANED OUT OF YOUR DIET**. You should also *stay away from the finely ground white flour breads* as these are nearly like eating candy or pastries.

If you are looking for more Calories to eliminate, look carefully at this group. First, eliminate the low-nutrition, high-Calorie foods. There are a *huge* number of these, and I have already pointed out many of them. When this is not enough, look at the other grain foods you eat. For example, you may eat a sandwich using two slices of bread or eat two slices of toast with your breakfast. Reduce your Calories by cutting back to one slice of bread for your sandwich or toast. You may also look for high-quality bread with fewer Calories per slice and continue to eat two slices. If you eat bread for every meal, you may try skipping bread with some of your meals or eat a smaller portion such as a half slice. Another option would be to eat rolled oats or cracked wheat for a cereal-grains serving.

Strive to eat bread made from the most coarsely ground flour. There is a wide variety of these available. The catch-22 here is that bread makers tend to throw in a lot of extra ingredients to make their bread a little tastier than the next, resulting in higher-Calorie breads. Most of your cereal-grains group will eventually be from coarsely ground whole-grain breads or whole-grain cereals.

Eating appropriately from this group will not be as easy as eating fruits and vegetables because cereal grains are contained in so many food items. However, **IT IS POSSIBLE WHEN YOU LEARN TO EAT THE LEAST-PROCESSED FOODS AVAILABLE**.

Fruits

On the food pyramid, it is suggested that you eat two to four servings of fruit daily. For example, you may eat an apple or orange per day but also eat a bunch of grapes and a peach or pear. These are your two to four servings of fruit. If you are looking for a way to reduce your Calories in the fruit group, only eat one apple, peach, pear, or orange per day. It is okay to throw in a few grapes or berries or similar fruits that are small in volume. There are differences in the caloric content of the different fruits. Just look up the number of Calories for the ones that you are not sure about.

You may also notice that you only eat these five types of fruit. Expand your variety by adding pineapple (fresh if at all possible; canned fruit has a lot of added sugar that you don't need), banana, kiwi, apricot, grapefruit, guava, papaya, melon, a wide variety of berries such as raspberries, strawberries, blueberries, blackberries, huckleberries, boysenberries, and many other fruits.

Now you have a much-bigger selection to choose from. However, *you only need to eat one or two types of fruit per day.* As your list of fruits enlarges, you may eat a particular fruit only once or twice per week. Also, there may be fruits that are only readily available during certain times of the year, such as raspberries, loganberries, chokecherries, etc. Take advantage of these fruits when they are available, and if possible, **STORE SOME FOR OFF-SEASON USE**. *Freeze them* as this does not require adding extra sugar and better preserves their natural nutrients and flavor. Note that some fruits do not freeze well such as peaches. These need to be preserved by other methods.

Protein

As you move up the food pyramid, notice that the quantity of food you eat from the groups gets smaller. This group is very important for supplying amino acids, iron, saturated fats, and other nutritional components needed in smaller quantities. *You should not skip this group to keep your Calories down. Instead, learn to get the necessary nutritional components without consuming too many Calories.*

For example, red meat is a valuable source of protein and iron, but it is also a source for larger quantities of fat. Eating red meat daily may give you a high-caloric intake that is difficult to overcome due to the excess fat. Rather than eliminating this option, only eat it once or twice per week with a smaller portion. Try eating more white meat such as chicken or turkey, or eat more fish or seafood to reduce your caloric input from this group. Eat more leafy green vegetables to enhance your iron intake.

Also, *people tend to overcook their meats,* especially red meat and poultry. Bear in mind that cooking any meat to well-done destroys a large portion of the protein content. Heaven forbid that you should eat meat that has a little pink tinge to it. Try to eat your red meat without charcoaling it (that is, cooking it until it is brown throughout) to better preserve the protein content.

There are fewer tendencies to overcook white meat or fish, except for chicken and turkey. *It is more common for poultry to contain bacteria,* but any type of meat or other food source could be contaminated. Health officials recommend heating poultry to a certain temperature to kill the bacteria, thereby preventing illness. However, *more of the amino acids are destroyed by these high temperatures. By eating a wider variety of meat, especially those that aren't recommended to be prepared at high temperatures, you will get a better complement of amino acids.*

As **YOUR BODY NEEDS PROTEIN FOR ESSENTIALLY**

EVERY FUNCTION AND EVERY TISSUE, your protein needs are relatively high. This does not mean that you need to consume large quantities of meat. A typical American diet usually contains a much higher-protein composition than needed for good health. Remember that many vegetables, grains, and dairy also contain protein.

Meat is going to put the capstone on protein to ensure adequate intake, so don't overdo it. Also *remember that eggs are an excellent protein source,* so if you eat eggs, your protein intake should be adequate. Try to keep the portions relative to other food groups as suggested by the food pyramids, and you will do fine.

By the way, **YOU DO NOT NEED TO USE SUPPLEMENTAL PROTEINS EVEN IF YOU WORK OUT VERY INTENSELY**. This is just another unnecessary caloric intake where promoters take advantage of your ignorance. Just consuming large quantities of protein is not going to make your muscles bigger. However, it may make you fatter by consuming extra, unnecessary Calories.

Dairy

The recommended number of servings for dairy is 1 to 2. The main thing to eat is **BUTTER**. If you eat butter and use some of the other components on a daily basis, you will get the nutrition available from dairy. *This is an important food group, so don't shy away from it.* If you like to drink milk for every meal, go ahead and do it. You may want to use 2 percent milk and/or cut down on the volume to help with caloric intake. Also, *eating cheese, cottage cheese, yogurt, etc., supplies everything that reduced fat milk does,* so if you eat from these other components and don't drink milk, that is okay. Many people do not eat milk products except for cheese. You need to work some of the other milk products into your diet (especially butter) to ensure the best nutritional benefit from this group.

Also remember that *many products like yogurt have a large amount of sugar added* to make it palatable (depending on the yogurt). Therefore, if you are looking for a place to reduce Calories from dairy without compromising its nutritional components, cut out portions that have added

Calories such as those found in yogurt. *Read the nutritional labels if you are unsure of the composition of the product, and avoid those with added sugar.*

You may be saying to yourself that you cannot eat dairy as you have lactose intolerance. *Unless you have not been able to eat dairy from birth, it is unlikely that you are truly lactose intolerant.* The intolerance comes about from not eating dairy. Over time, the cells in your digestive tract that produce lactase, the enzyme necessary to metabolize the lactose in milk products, lose their ability to readily produce this enzyme. Therefore, when you eat lactose, it does not get digested and stimulates your bowels, resulting in gas production and high motility. You then pass large amounts of gas with diarrhea and possibly some cramping.

To regain your ability to digest lactose, start by eating a very small portion of dairy such as a sip of milk or a small spoon of yogurt or ice cream. Do this every day, increasing the amount you eat slightly. Over time, you will regain your ability to produce lactase in sufficient quantities to digest dairy appropriately. (It is a similar story with prunes as they contain a complex sugar that is hard to digest for the same reason that lactose is. Eating prunes daily will allow you to eat them without causing diarrhea.)

Combination Foods

Most likely, you are not going to just eat individual items from the five food groups. You will combine several ingredients from various groups to make a particular dish. This could be anything from a sandwich to a very complex baked entrée. *Consider the ingredients from the various groups represented in the recipe as part of the servings for that group.* For example, you make a sandwich for lunch. You use coarsely ground multigrain bread, roasted turkey, cheddar cheese, spinach, and tomatoes. This represents servings from the cereal grains, protein, dairy, and vegetable groups.

ADDITIONAL PHYSIOLOGICAL FACTS

I have already addressed several physiological functions in previous sections. This section will address some additional **IMPORTANT INFORMATION** that you need to understand. Most people are aware of the facts that I address in this section. They are self-evident but apparently very hard to understand.

Your Body Cannot Generate Mass from Nothing

This is probably the most important fact that you need to get a good grasp on and not forget. **YOUR BODY IS INCAPABLE OF GENERATING MUSCLE, BONE, FAT, SKIN, OR ANY OTHER TYPE OF TISSUE, WITHOUT HAVING THE NECESSARY COMPONENTS SUPPLIED THROUGH YOUR DIET**.

One thing that I hear very frequently is patients (and many other people) complaining about not being able to lose weight. They say they eat very little and don't understand how they cannot lose weight. I try to explain in a nice way that they are simply eating too much, but usually they insist that they do not overeat and need some medication that will allow them to lose weight. This is most distressing to me as I do not have sufficient time to discuss the facts with them, and they don't understand their bodies well enough to know that mass cannot be generated from nothing. They leave my office with their false belief still intact, and I feel terrible as I have not been able to appropriately help them.

Now you are probably already thinking about Aunt Harriet, who has a medical problem and is taking medicine that caused her to gain a lot of weight and swell up like a balloon, and you know that she almost eats nothing. There are several medical conditions that interfere with metabolic function and slow down your metabolism (the rate you consume or use energy). An individual whose thyroid does not produce enough hormones is one example. People, like Aunt Harriet, who are on catabolic steroids experience several interferences of their body's functions, some of which cause them to retain water that causes the swelling and weight gain.

If any of these people stop eating, they *will lose weight.* **IT IS IMPOSSIBLE FOR ANYONE TO EAT NOTHING AND GAIN WEIGHT.** If they drink water, they may temporarily gain weight from water retention but will then lose weight as their body starts to consume itself to provide energy for its basic metabolism and sheds the excess water.

Calories In, Calories Out

Signs with this information are posted at some gyms and many other locations. These seem to be self-evident principles but also do not seem to be understood. This may be because people think that these principles do not apply to them. Just like the patient who states that he or she eats almost nothing but still gains weight and needs diet pills or some other assistance to lose weight must think that these principles do not apply to him or her. **GET THIS FACT FIRMLY PLANTED IN YOUR HEAD**. *If you are dieting but not losing weight,* **YOU ARE SIMPLY EATING TOO MANY CALORIES FOR YOUR NEEDS**.

You may be eating inappropriately. For example, if you live on fast foods or processed foods such as potato chips, candy, pop, cake, pasta, and many other foods, you will find that a small portion has a lot of Calories. Therefore, without realizing it, you will be overeating. When eating healthy foods such as vegetables, fruits, lean meat, etc., it is surprising how much you can eat before consuming the same number of Calories. *In fact, you probably could not eat the volume of healthy food that is equal to the number of Calories contained in the unhealthy food you eat.*

Your current lifestyle, physical condition, or medical condition may not allow you to eat very many Calories without severely overeating. Remember that if you do nothing but lie on the couch and watch TV, you can still lose weight if you eat the appropriate number of Calories. This may be a very small amount of food, depending on the type of food, but it's still possible.

At this point, you may doubt everything I have said. You may be saying to yourself, "I know that this is not true as I have dieted very seriously and not lost any weight. Therefore, this guy is full of $@&# and doesn't know what he is talking about. I must have a medical problem preventing me from losing weight." In this case, you may have a medical problem called denial. *If you understand that your body cannot generate mass from nothing, you must realize that* **IT IS IMPOSSIBLE FOR YOU TO NOT LOSE WEIGHT IF YOU EAT APPROPRIATELY.** You may not be able to eat very much, but *if you eat appropriately for your metabolic needs, you will lose weight.*

Use of Food Components

Some people (a lot of people and even a lot of educated people) think that your body uses the various components of the food you eat such as proteins, carbohydrates, cartilage, and others just the way they are contained in the food. *The facts are that the proteins and other molecules used by your body are very different from those found in the things you eat.* Of course, you don't usually eat other humans. *Even if you did, your body would still have to break down the proteins and other molecules into basic components before your body could use them.* Between individuals, many of the molecules used for the same function are slightly different. As evidence of this, people respond differently to the same medication. For example, the antihistamine Benadryl (diphenhydramine) causes most people to be very sleepy. However, it makes some people hyperactive.

The various components of your food are broken down into their basic building blocks and even smaller molecules and atoms. From the information on protein, you learned that proteins are made up of building blocks called amino acids. As dietary protein is digested, it is broken down into the amino acid building blocks. These are then used to manufacture all the various proteins your body needs. The proteins they come from are immaterial.

Another example of a misconception is the ingestion of cartilage or portions of cartilage to improve your joint health. Special cells make the cartilage in your joints and other areas of your body. *The basic building blocks for cartilage are found in many foods.* Therefore, eating additional portions of cartilage *does not* help your body improve joint health. Also, taking one of several supplements that come with many combinations of molecules found in cartilage such as glucosamine, chondroitin, methylsulfonylmethane, hyaluronic acid, and other molecules from various herbs is **NOT NECESSARY** for good joint health.

If you have noticed an improvement after taking one of these supplements, it is because **YOUR DIET IS DEFICIENT IN PROVIDING THE NECESSARY NUTRITIONAL COMPONENTS** that your body needs to maintain your joints, and *the supplement merely provides those components.* You may have just experienced a placebo effect. (By the way, you cannot digest cartilage—it just passes straight through.)

EATING A HEALTHY DIET IS MUCH MORE IMPORTANT THAN TRYING TO TAKE SPECIAL SUPPLEMENTS TO ENHANCE CERTAIN FUNCTIONS OF YOUR BODY. Your body utilizes building blocks contained in a good diet to produce the various molecules and tissues required for proper body functioning. If your diet is deficient in certain required components, the part of your body that needs those components as building blocks will not function properly.

Drink According to Your Thirst

This statement is going to raise a lot of controversy, but only among those who embrace the **"NEED TO DRINK A SPECIFIC AMOUNT OF WATER DAILY" FALLACY.**

Water is an area that is highly misunderstood and very much exploited. Somewhere, someone started promoting the myth that we need to drink large quantities of water daily. It was probably the nutritionist who, many years ago, started promoting drinking eight eight-ounce glasses of water daily. Although the information was completely unfounded, it caught on and became popular. It has since been proven that this idea is not true, but it has been difficult to change everyone's thinking. (Once you start a boulder rolling downhill, it is very hard to stop.)

The trend was popular for a while and then died down, until bottled water came on the scene, when drinking a specific amount of water daily suddenly became popular again. Water is an important component of your body as it composes approximately 70 percent of it. There is water inside each cell, surrounding each cell, in your cardiovascular system (veins and arteries), fluid surrounding your brain and spinal cord, etc. This water is used for a number of functions but is most obviously used to carry molecules throughout your body (nutrients necessary for cellular function) and to carry by-products of metabolism (waste products) to your kidneys, lungs, and liver for expulsion.

We do need to drink a certain amount daily, but **THE EXACT AMOUNT IS DEPENDENT ON MANY VARIABLES.** How big is your body? What is the temperature outside? How active have you been? Have you just been lying around, watching TV, or working hard outside in the sun? People make claims like "You have to drink three quarts of water daily in order for your body to properly flush itself of harmful chemicals, toxins, and metabolic by-products."

The plain fact is, your body is designed to excrete chemicals, toxins, and metabolic by-products under a variety of hydration states. Additionally, *sludge does not build up in your body like sludge in your car's engine.* Your body does not have little nooks and crannies for by-products to build up in. Therefore, you **CANNOT** wash them out by drinking more water to flush your system.

Another claim is that diluting the pollutants (metabolic by-products or undesired ingested chemicals) will decrease their effect on your body. Chemical reactions are dependent on the concentration of chemicals that are interacting with one another. However, *the overall effect of you diluting the chemicals and your body reconcentrating them is the same as if you maintained a normal hydration state.*

Your body eliminates and deactivates undesired chemicals by the following processes. As your blood returns from the various parts of your body, ALL your blood is accumulated into a common vessel and routed to your heart. ALL your blood is then pumped through your lungs, where metabolic by-products (carbon dioxide) can be exchanged for oxygen. Your body's needs for oxygen and elimination of carbon dioxide are great enough at times that it requires the maximum capacity of your lungs to provide this exchange. For example, athletes performing at their peak need all the oxygen they can get and elimination of all the carbon dioxide produced from their muscle activity. All your blood then returns to your heart, where it is pumped to the remainder of your body.

The remainder of your metabolic by-products (waste) does not occur in sufficient quantities that it requires the constant elimination of 100 percent of those by-products. A large percentage of your blood flows through your liver, but a much-smaller portion actually flows through your kidneys. The kidneys clean that portion of your blood, and when it returns to the rest of the circulation, it dilutes the remaining by-products to keep them at tolerable levels.

This is done by allowing the undesired by-products and many desired molecules to leave the kidney's circulatory system and enter the kidney filtration system. The filtration system then reabsorbs the desired molecules and lets the undesired molecules flow into the urine. If the blood is more concentrated, meaning that there is less water circulating, more of the undesired chemicals are excreted per volume of circulating blood. If the blood is more dilute, the undesired chemicals are also less concentrated, and fewer of them are excreted per volume of blood processed by the kidneys.

WHEN YOU DRINK WATER, YOUR BODY IS OBLIGATED TO ABSORB IT INTO YOUR CIRCULATION (it has to be absorbed; your body cannot choose whether or not to absorb the water). If you have too much water in your circulatory system, specific molecules that the kidneys monitor are too dilute. The kidneys will then excrete more water in order to bring the concentration of these molecules back to normal. Some of the excess water may seep into tissue, causing swelling. **THE OVERALL NET EFFECT FROM DILUTING AND THEN RECONCENTRATING YOUR BLOOD IS EXCRETION OF THE SAME AMOUNT OF BY-PRODUCTS OVER A PERIOD OF TIME.** Drinking more water *does not* result in a decrease in the amount of circulating by-products; it only temporarily dilutes them. The main result of drinking more water is more frequent trips to the bathroom, especially at night.

I have rarely heard the argument that drinking more water will reduce the incidence of kidney stones (which are crystals of various components of urine). The formation of stones only occurs when certain molecules exist in sufficient concentration. There are several types made up of molecules of metabolism and from dietary sources. Some people are more genetically prone to developing kidney stones. However, in virtually all cases, stones are not a problem if you remain adequately hydrated. This does not mean consuming large volumes of water. **IT MEANS DRINKING ACCORDING TO YOUR THIRST.**

As with the kidneys, it is not necessary for the liver to detoxify 100 percent of the toxins in your blood on a continual basis. When the toxins are dilute, your liver detoxifies fewer of them per volume of blood. Similarly, when your blood is concentrated, more of the toxins are detoxified. The net result is the same.

THE ONLY WAY THAT WASTE OR TOXINS BECOME A FACTOR IS WHEN THERE IS A PERSISTENT DEHYDRATION STATE OR EXCESSIVE INGESTION OR PRODUCTION OF THESE HARMFUL PRODUCTS. In these situations, your liver may not be able to keep up with detoxification and your kidneys with elimination. Therefore, metabolic waste and toxin concentration could exist at high-enough levels to cause problems with metabolic functions. However, consuming excessive water is not going to solve the problem. Maintaining adequate hydration will prevent dehydration from being an issue. You need to avoid as much exposure to the harmful chemicals as possible and correct the abnormal production of them, which could be dietary or genetic. Eating a proper diet will correct the dietary production. A genetic disorder will have to be handled by other means.

YOUR BODY IS VERY GOOD AT TELLING YOU WHEN TO DRINK AND HOW MUCH. Just think of the various situations that may exist during a particular day and at various times of the year. For example, someone working outside in the summer may require more than a gallon or two of water during the day to accommodate the fluid lost from sweating and urinating (and other functions such as breathing). The same person who works in an air-conditioned office, drives in an air-conditioned car, and lives in an air-conditioned house may only need a quart of water to maintain the same hydration state. Also, there would be a huge difference in water needs between a ninety-pound person and a three-hundred-pound person under the same conditions. **IT IS IMPOSSIBLE TO ACCURATELY PREDICT HOW MUCH EACH OF THESE INDIVIDUALS WOULD NEED TO BE NORMALLY HYDRATED.**

Researchers have looked into the high-water-intake issue. Their findings indicate that your body really does NOT need a specified amount of fluid intake per day (such as eight eight-ounce glasses) but **ONLY THE AMOUNT NECESSARY TO SATISFY YOUR THIRST**. If you pay attention to your thirst and treat it appropriately, you will supply your body with just the right amount of fluid. Just like how you don't have to control your breathing or heart rate, your body knows best how much fluid you need. The difference is, when your body tells you it needs more fluid, you do have to provide that fluid. It cannot obtain it without your help.

There are many sources giving you information on how to calculate your daily water requirements. **DON'T RELY ON SOME FORMULA OR SOMEONE SELLING YOU BOTTLED WATER TO TELL YOU HOW MUCH TO DRINK. RELY ON YOUR BODY TO TELL YOU HOW MUCH WATER YOU NEED.**

WHY ISN'T MY DIET WORKING?

You now have the necessary information on physiology and nutrition you need to eat healthily. I have also given information enabling you to understand why all the diet programs, medications, herbs, supplements, and natural medicines are all fallacies. Now that you know the extent that the supplement and diet industries have gone to promote products and programs for financial gain, we need to explore why people fail at losing weight and then look at ways to avoid those failures.

Most people, at some time in their life, have tried some program to lose weight. Diets, supplements, herbs, medications, exercise programs, etc., are all lumped under program for the remainder of this book. Almost without exception, **EVERYONE HAS REGAINED THE UNWANTED WEIGHT WITH USUALLY A LITTLE EXTRA**. *Why do people keep failing at their attempts to lose weight? The problem is inherent in* **BASIC HUMAN NATURE,** *not some magic program.*

For example, certain activities provide stress relief. Frequently, one of these is eating. After a hard day at work, or especially at home with the kids, you like to sit down with your favorite beverage or snack and watch a little TV or listen to music or whatever. While at work, you look forward to your little break, where you eat your Twinkies and drink your soda pop. When you sit down to that bowl of pasta for your evening meal (I only use pasta as an example; there are many high-Calorie comfort foods), you feel gratified as the succulent noodles with the rich creamy cheese sauce slide down your throat. Afterward, you feel fulfilled and satisfied. You may be the type that as the late-evening news begins, you get a bowl of your favorite ice cream and enjoy it as you watch the news.

The usual outcome is that **OVER TIME, YOU END UP OVERWEIGHT**. Distraught with your current condition, you seek a method to correct the problem. Not knowing where to turn, you remember the ads that you saw on television or the Internet or heard on the radio. You may even consult your friends for advice. Just as bad (or probably worse), you may go to a physician for advice. What you usually end up with is some program designed to help you lose weight.

You follow the program, and sure enough, you lose weight. However, you are miserable the entire time, having to forgo your rituals and probably completely changing your diet and/or lifestyle in order to reduce your caloric intake sufficiently to lose weight. However, you persist as you know that in a short time, you will reach your promised goal. Once achieved, you can finally return to your greatly missed rituals. There are several fallacies in this scenario:

1) To start with, the people who come up with these programs have something in it for themselves. I don't mean to suggest that they do anything dishonest. I am sure they think they have discovered the key to the obesity problem and hope to make a profit while helping those who use their program. **ALL THE PROGRAMS ARE FLAWED** and fall short of what you really need. They all work some angle, suggesting that you should only eat carbohydrates or proteins or use certain compounds that they have concocted to lose weight. Some programs even provide food for you.

   THEY FAIL TO ADDRESS THE REAL ISSUES OF GOOD HEALTH THROUGH PROPER NUTRITION in a way that doesn't require their support. Also, **YOU DON'T LEARN TO EAT IN A WAY THAT IS SATISFYING TO YOU,** is nutritious, and can be maintained for a lifetime. Most plans claim that their program is nutritionally sound although virtually none of them are. Another thing in common is that they **ALL FORCE YOU TO REDUCE YOUR CALORIC INTAKE TO SUFFICIENT LEVELS TO CAUSE RAPID WEIGHT LOSS** (or at least guarantee weight loss). They know that people are impatient and want to achieve their weight goals immediately: no time to wait; get that weight off now!

These programs fail to acknowledge the issues of lifelong changes that require a certain amount of time to accomplish. Their approach is to appeal to the urgency to lose weight quickly and take advantage of the ignorance of the people embracing their programs.

2) The people who recommend these programs to you (including physicians) know little if anything about weight loss and maintaining your desired weight. Additionally, they know less about nutrition, which is not even addressed. Their information comes from diet plans, radio, television, their family physician, newspapers, other friends, etc. They may have even tried one or several of these programs and found success in a particular one. Now they are recommending it to you.

3) If you consulted your physician, you may be in for a bigger surprise. I don't think that it was stated any better than by an author who wrote a nutrition book in the 1970s: what most physicians know about nutrition, they learned from another physician, who heard it from someone else. In other words, physicians do not have the time to spend on nutrition that would help them become proficient in giving good advice (this includes diet programs, supplements, herbs, etc.). It was true then and is certainly true now: there are too many other things physicians need to learn. There is simply not enough time to incorporate a significant amount of nutrition into a medical curriculum. The physicians who do know something about nutrition or weight loss have learned it from independent study. Also, **THE APPROACH MEDICINE IS TAKING TOWARD THE OBESITY PROBLEM DEMONSTRATES A CLEAR MISUNDERSTANDING OF THE MAJOR ISSUES ASSOCIATED WITH OBESITY**. Heaven forbid that a physician should actually admit that he or she doesn't really know very much about these things and refer you to someone who may know (it is unlikely that they know someone who could truly help you).

Also, **IF YOU KNOW A LOT ABOUT NUTRITION, IT DOES NOT NECESSARILY HELP YOU KNOW HOW TO CONTROL YOUR WEIGHT**. If this were true, all nutritionists would have an appropriate weight and maximize their health, and everyone who followed their advice would be the same. When you look around, it is obvious that this is not true. *There is much more to dieting (eating properly) and maintaining a desired weight than just knowing what foods are good for you.*

Diet pills are the worst. There are many approaches to diet pills. Your body is a finely tuned machine, and science certainly does not have the knowledge to improve the way it functions. Therefore, any attempts to alter your body's functions are fraught with problems.

Actually, diet pills are not the worst way to lose weight; **HAVING SURGERY IS.** It does not alter the way you have to eat to be healthy and lose weight. You may temporarily lose weight as you eat the diet prescribed by the surgeon. However, once you recover from the surgery, you still have to eat appropriately to keep losing weight or maintain your weight. You can gain a large amount of weight by eating frequent small amounts of high-Calorie foods.

4) By whatever means you manage to lose your weight, you have not succeeded in **PERMANENTLY** changing your lifestyle sufficiently to maintain your desired weight. Once you meet your short-term goal, which is your targeted weight, you have two options. One is to continue with the program you are using. In this case, you are probably nutritionally deficient, as it is unlikely that the program is nutritionally sound, and frustrated because you cannot pursue your previous diet. The other option is to return to your long-awaited snacks and favorite foods that you so sorely missed. Returning to them is, of course, pursuing the things that made you fat in the first place. Now that you have returned to them, you can expect to get fat again just like you did before. The downside is that you usually gain back more weight than what you lost during your dieting fiasco.

Another fact is, **MOST PEOPLE NEVER REACH THEIR DESIRED WEIGHT**. Along the way, they experience too much stress over loss of their previous favorite foods and slowly or quickly start to slip back into them. After spending a sufficient amount of frustrating time pursuing a program while slipping in and out of their old diet, they give up and continue with their old diet without ever reaching their target weight.

You can see that **FOLLOWING ANY PROGRAM CAN LEAD TO WEIGHT LOSS**. It is very easy to lose weight. Just don't eat, and you will lose weight. This is the fastest weight-loss plan, but it is also the least-healthy approach and would lead to the greatest rebound weight gain. **ALL THE PROGRAMS FORCE YOU TO REDUCE YOUR CALORIC INTAKE SUFFICIENTLY TO RESULT IN WEIGHT LOSS**. Most of them are not nutritionally sound and do not result in lifelong dietary changes that are necessary if you are to maintain your weight and especially your health. **IT IS IMPORTANT TO GET THESE IDEAS FIRMLY PLANTED IN YOUR MIND**.

Habits

HUMANS ARE CREATURES OF HABIT. Virtually everything is done on a habitual basis. The way you walk, brush your teeth, comb your hair, sleep, put on your clothes, and do many other things are all done habitually. **THIS INCLUDES WHAT YOU EAT, WHEN YOU EAT, WHERE YOU EAT, AND WHY YOU EAT.**

In the examples at the beginning of the last section, several scenarios were described where you eat comfort food. Having enjoyed your favorite food ritual, you are now ready to move on to the next activity for the day. **THIS LITTLE RITUAL BECOMES A HABIT**—a very powerful habit. If you are not allowed to carry out this routine, you experience much discomfort (stress or anxiety). There are many other scenarios that result in the development of powerful habits with your snacking and mealtime choices.

Habits seem to be easy to start but can be **EXTREMELY DIFFICULT TO CHANGE OR STOP**. For example, you start drinking a beverage during break at work. Soon, you will not be able to take that break without drinking the beverage. You start looking forward to the break, and being deprived of this opportunity causes you to feel anxiety that is relieved by the consumption of the beverage. To stop this habit takes significant effort, and some people never stop.

One of the most powerful habits is cigarette smoking. It takes a surprisingly few episodes to initiate an intense habit. Most everyone is aware of the difficulty of quitting smoking even if they have never smoked. Is it because of the powerful nicotine addiction? No, it is because of the **POWERFUL HABITUAL ADDICTION.** Although this section is about diets, the habitual addiction is the same. Since most people have a sense of how difficult it is for smokers to quit, it may be easier to understand the eating addiction by reviewing a little bit about the better-understood addiction of smoking.

Cigarette-smoking addiction comes in two parts. One is the addiction to nicotine. As with most drug-induced addictions, the addiction comes from the need to avoid withdrawal symptoms. (Another addictive drive comes from the need to experience euphoria. Euphoria is not part of this addiction and plays a minimal role compared to the withdrawal symptoms.) When a cigarette smoker goes too long without a cigarette, he or she may start to get jittery, anxious, nervous and possibly experience a headache, stomach cramps, or other symptoms. Smoking provides the nicotine that relieves these symptoms, releasing the anxiety caused by them. *If this were the only addiction from smoking, it would be easy to overcome by using nicotine in other forms.*

The fact is that few (if any) smokers are actually helped by taking nicotine. This is because most of them are not addicted to it. Therefore, they experience no withdrawal symptoms or at least very minimal ones. **THE MOST INTENSE SYMPTOMS** (anxiety) **COME FROM THE HABITUAL ACT OF SMOKING THE CIGARETTE.** Usually, smokers have several situations where they enjoy smoking. This may be after a meal, while driving a car, when taking a break at work, or when feeling stressed from a variety of causes. The smoker is usually looking forward to smoking that cigarette either *consciously* or *subconsciously*. If the act of smoking cannot be carried out, *anxiety* starts to build, increasing the desire to smoke. For those addicted to nicotine, the anxiety is intensified by the withdrawal symptoms that are occurring from the lack of nicotine.

Breaking a habit is not an easy thing to do. This is evident by the great number of self-help books written on how to break habits. Many approaches have been presented, and success in breaking or changing habits has been variable. This is because if you **ABRUPTLY CHANGE A HABIT** (or keep yourself from engaging in the habit), you usually experience such **EXTREME ANXIETY THAT YOU CANNOT CONTINUE AVOIDING THE HABIT.**

The anxiety can be suppressed for a while, from minutes to days, depending on the reason for suppressing the urge. I have seen women go their entire pregnancy without smoking to avoid exposing the baby to complications caused from cigarette smoke. Most, if not all of them, return to smoking, from immediately after the baby is born to several days to even weeks after the birth. Smokers will tell you, "It is easy to quit smoking. I have done it a thousand times." What they are really saying is "I can suppress the urge and, thus, the anxiety to smoke for a while," but the anxiety will eventually override their willpower to resist, and they will smoke again. This behavior is not unique to smokers, alcoholics, and drug addicts. It is also noted in individuals who have other addictive behaviors. Remember, **TO SUCCESSFULLY CHANGE ANY HABIT, YOU MUST LEARN HOW TO DEAL WITH THIS ANXIETY IN A WAY THAT WILL ALLOW YOU TO BE SUCCESSFUL.**

Dieting Habits

Most people have developed habits in their eating patterns that have led them to being overweight. The altering of these habits is no different from a person trying to quit smoking. The **DENIAL** of that snack-time treat, that bowl of ice cream, or that favorite pasta dish produces an **ANXIETY** that results in eating the treat, ice cream, or pasta to relieve the anxiety. Just like the smoker, the anxiety may be suppressed for a while, but sooner or later (usually sooner), the urge will win out, and the person will satisfy the anxiety by eating the desired food.

Similar to smoking, there may be chemicals in food that cause certain feelings when that particular food is not eaten. However, like nicotine, *these feelings are inconsequential when compared to your eating habits.*

Just like smoking, **IF YOU CANNOT ENGAGE IN YOUR EATING HABITS, ANXIETY STARTS TO BUILD UNTIL YOU SATISFY IT**.

This is what happens to people on diet plans. They develop such strong urges to return to their old eating habits that they keep slipping in and out of their diet plan until they finally give up and go back to their old eating habits. I suppose most people could say, "I can diet anytime I want. I have done it a thousand times." Therefore, the problem that you must first face when trying to lose weight is **LEARNING TO DEAL WITH THE ANXIETY CAUSED BY THE CHANGE IN YOUR EATING HABITS.**

When engaging in a diet plan, there is **NO THOUGHT OF CONTROLLING THE EATING ANXIETY.** There is only the desire to not be fat anymore. The anxiety is felt but not understood. The thought *I can endure this change in my diet for a time to lose the weight* is strong enough to allow you to initiate your diet plan. This works for various lengths of time before you give in to your anxiety and resume your previous eating habits. This may take a few days or even weeks, but eventually, you will return to your old eating habits where you find comfort. This may even be after you attain your weight goals.

THE MOST IMPORTANT ASPECT OF A SUCCESSFUL DIET PLAN IS TO OVERCOME THE HABITS THAT YOU HAVE FOR HIGH-CALORIE, LOW-NUTRITION FOOD, ENGAGING IN A FAVORITE SNACK-TIME TREAT AND INDULGING IN LARGE QUANTITIES OF FOOD. Remember, when you develop eating habits, they include the types of food you eat, the amount that you eat, and the timing of when you eat meals or snacks.

Of course, there are times when you cannot pacify a habit such as when you attend a party, go to a movie, or other similar event. However, your desire is masked by that activity, so you don't miss it as greatly. Also, you know that you can still have the food item any time you want. You are not being deprived of it or denying yourself; you are simply *postponing* it.

You should now see that the **ANXIETY** that occurs when you make any life change is the limiting factor in being successful at maintaining that change. There are many situations where this type of anxiety could occur such as **BREAKING ANY HABIT,** engaging in some **DIETING PROGRAM,** learning to eat healthily, learning to exercise appropriately, finding a new job, moving to a new city, etc. **THE KEY FOR SUCCESS IS FOR YOU TO RECOGNIZE AND DEAL WITH THIS ANXIETY APPROPRIATELY**. *It is amazing to me that research, including that performed by the medical community, fails to address this most basic factor of obesity.* Subsequent sections will explore ways to successfully deal with this anxiety.

Morbid Obesity and Psychiatric Disorders

Special consideration may be given to people who are morbidly obese (BMI of ~35+ or more than 1.5 times their normal body weight). Some of these people have more of an eating disorder rather than just habitual eating. Their disorder often has a depression component or possibly an obsessive-compulsive component. The depressed person is more likely to eat to treat his or her depression. Eating brings relief of the depression. It gives a feeling of comfort and pleasure that doesn't seem to be available from any other source. The obsessive-compulsive person needs to eat to relieve the anxiety from his or her disorder. Another disorder causing excessive weight gain is the binge-eating disorder.

The addition of unrelated psychiatric disorders to the usual eating anxiety may make it very difficult for these individuals to lose weight. They may need some kind of pharmacological help in the way of antianxiety or antidepression medication and/or counseling. People who have these disorders are typically dysfunctional in other ways, which results in them being diagnosed and treated for their condition independently of their weight problem.

The difficulty for them is being able to change their eating habits in any fashion that will bring about the permanent changes necessary to meet their weight and health goals. The maintenance of their comfort level due to their psychological disorder is much more important than losing weight. There are very few people who would have these disorders compared to the number who are overweight. To even function at any level in life, they usually need some kind of help in the way of counseling and/or medication.

I only bring this topic up because I know some people use the excuse that they have some other disorder preventing them from losing weight. However, it is more likely that either they won't admit that they have to change the way they eat to lose weight or they are not willing to put out the effort it will require to make these life changes. They will insist that they have a problem that makes them gain weight, or are on some medication that makes them gain weight. But there is nothing that is going to make them gain weight. Some medications and physical conditions may make it difficult to lose weight, but not impossible.

There are some people in this category whose **WEIGHT IS THE CAUSE** of their depression or other related psychological disorder. They may require counseling to help them deal with eating or realize that they eat to treat their feelings about their obesity. Usually, their attempts to use fad diets, supplements, etc., have met with failure, leaving them little hope that there is a way for them to lose their weight and have a normal lifestyle.

Surgical Weight Loss

You may also be considering surgery to achieve your weight goals. This is, of course, an extreme measure to achieve **SELF-CONTROL**. The surgery will, at first, force you to change your eating habits. It may cause you to get a full sensation after eating a small amount. Nausea and vomiting may occur if you eat too much. **IF YOU DON'T LEARN TO EAT APPROPRIATELY, YOU WILL GAIN BACK ANY WEIGHT LOST AND MAY BE IN WORSE HEALTH SECONDARY TO ANY BOWEL DISTURBANCE AFFECTING NUTRIENT-ABSORBING SURFACES.**

The medical benefits, such as reduction in diabetes, blood pressure, etc., which are claimed to come about because of surgical procedures, are actually due to the **CHANGES IN DIET** required after the surgery **AND THE ASSOCIATED WEIGHT LOSS.** These same dietary changes can be made without going through the surgery. **SO THE REAL BENEFITS COME FROM DIETARY CHANGES, NOT FROM SURGERY.**

So what's it going to be: **SURGERY WITH THE COINCIDENT NEED TO LEARN TO EAT APPROPRIATELY** OR **JUST**

LEARNING TO EAT APPROPRIATELY? I know several people who have taken both roads. The majority of those having surgery gained most or all their weight back with a little added bonus of additional weight, and some developed malabsorption problems. Most of the ones who achieved their weight goals by learning to eat appropriately are still maintaining their desired weight. Why? Because **IN ANY DIETARY PLAN, YOU HAVE TO COMMIT TO LIFELONG EATING CHANGES TO MAINTAIN YOUR DESIRED WEIGHT, REGARDLESS OF ANY OTHER CRUTCH YOU MAY USE ALONG THE WAY.** The crutches will all go away at some point. If you have **NOT** learned to eat appropriately for your caloric needs, you **WILL** put the weight back on.

Consideration for the Extremely Obese

Special consideration may be needed for those people who are very morbidly obese (BMI of greater than or equal to 60 or 2.5 times their normal body weight). Some of these people are in such poor health that they may die if not treated aggressively with good nutrition and more rapid weight loss. These are *medical cases* and are not subject to any dietary plan other than lifesaving procedures. However, once they are stable enough, they need to pursue a less aggressive weight-reduction process and learn to eat appropriately.

FAMILY MATTERS

Obesity does not usually reside in one individual in a family. The family members typically have similar physiques. "Oh, look at the Smith family. They must have something wrong with their genes. They are all fat." *People learn to eat from their parents* (who learned to eat from their parents) in a family environment where everyone eats the same food, has access to the same snacks, and develops similar types of **EATING HABITS,** which is often the cause of their weight problem, **NOT THEIR GENES.**

Some members of that family may also be significantly different from the others. For example, one may be much leaner. This could be for a variety of reasons. Maybe they are uncomfortable being fat and watch what they eat more closely or get full after eating a small amount of food, or maybe they play sports that require that they have a leaner habitus. Conversely, there may be one member who is much heavier than the other family members because he or she engages in excessive snacking or indulging at mealtime. There is also the situation where one family member has a medical problem such as a thyroid or growth-hormone disorder. In these instances, if there is any question, the family member should have a medical evaluation.

It is **EXTREMELY DIFFICULT** for a single member of such a family to engage in any nutritional plan to lose weight, unless it is the **PARENTS** who take the initiative. Notice that I said *parents*. If only one parent or child desires to improve his or her health and lose weight, he or she will get opposition from the spouse or other family members. This is particularly true if radical changes are proposed by those desiring to change. The other members are perfectly happy (or seem to be content) being fat and desire no change in their current habits. Actually, they are probably not content at all but don't know where to turn for help to lose weight in a tolerable fashion.

If you are the only individual in your family who desires change, it will be more difficult to improve your nutritional health as you will not be able to control your food choices. However, you can *still improve your health and lose weight as outlined in this book.* You will just have to do the best you can with the limited options available until you can live on your own or succeed in making family-wide changes.

The first person in a family to pick up on the information in this book should introduce the ideas to the other members. If you understand the material in this book, you will be able to demonstrate to the other family members that all of them can be successful at obtaining a more desirable body weight. They will also be nutritionally healthy and can accomplish these things without stressful, expensive, radical life changes such as those proposed by diet and weight-loss programs.

Have each member of your family read this book, or read it together. As your family utilizes the ideas outlined in this book, they will start to see changes that they thought could never happen. They will feel and look better in a way that will result in lifelong changes and habits. **DON'T BE DISCOURAGED** by whatever family situation you may be involved with, even if you are the only one engaged in this program.

PREPARING FOR CHANGE

In addition to the information on diet programs, supplements, nutrition, and physiology, you now know why you fail in your attempts at weight loss**.** It is the **STRESS** from **CHANGES** in your **DIETING HABITS** that you must learn to deal with. In most cases, eating nutritiously is not part of your diet plan. However, you should at least be starting to understand that nutrition is a major part of your health. If you would like to know more about nutrition, there are plenty of good resources to explore. However, even if you have detailed knowledge of this information, it will **NOT** help you lose weight or improve your nutritional status.

The statement **"YOU ARE WHAT YOU EAT"** is a literal statement. When you eat junk food, don't expect your body to turn it into healthy nutrients. *Your body is designed to produce certain products from specific molecules contained in your diet.* If it does not have the correct ones, don't expect it to turn out the correct products. (If you feed cotton into a spinning loom, don't expect silk thread.) To be nutritionally fit, you will have to make good food choices. This may mean giving up your most treasured foods that, by the way, *are killing you.* This does not mean that you can never have a bowl of ice cream or a candy bar or other tasty but generally bad-for-you food, but they will become a minuscule part of your diet.

Weight loss can be achieved by eating the correct amount of nutritionally poor food. Similarly, weight gain may occur by eating excessive amounts of nutritionally sound food. **IF YOU ARE SOMEWHAT OVERWEIGHT BUT NUTRITIONALLY FIT, YOU ARE BETTER OFF THAN EATING NUTRITIONALLY POOR FOOD AND BEING AT YOUR DESIRED WEIGHT.**

LEARNING TO EAT CORRECTLY MAY TAKE MONTHS OR

YEARS, depending on how poorly you eat and how out of shape you are nutritionally and physically. You spend years getting fat and being out of shape. Don't expect to reverse all your bad habits and rid yourself of all your cravings in a few weeks or even months. Weight change will also be slow. So what if it takes you five years to get to your desired weight? This is the weight you will have for the rest of your life, and you will have conquered the lifestyle that made you fat. Most importantly, *if you learn to eat the best foods you have available, you will be at your best nutritional health.*

Before getting into changing your eating habits, there are a few other things you need to understand.

Lifelong Changes

As you make changes to your diet, they must be **LIFELONG CHANGES**. It should be apparent that you can **NEVER** revert to your previous habits. To do so would result in pursuing the things that caused your problem in the first place. This, of course, would defeat anything that you had done to control your weight and be healthier. *You must understand that you are changing what you eat to lose weight and to be healthy and to maintain your weight and health for the* **REST OF YOUR LIFE**.

Choices

There are plenty of people who, when confronted with making dietary changes, exclaim, "I already eat a healthy, well-balanced diet." *Well, if you do, why are you fat?* Obviously, you don't eat a proper diet, although you could be eating a healthy diet. If you are one of those people who think they are already eating a healthy, proper diet but cannot lose weight because they have something else wrong with them, guess again. Reassess your diet, regroup, and start again. You are undoubtedly eating too many Calories for your needs.

Don't kid yourself into thinking that you already eat healthily. If you *do not* eat a variety from *all* the five major food groups (see Appendix 1) in the proper amounts and few, if any, processed foods, *your diet may be lacking in some important nutritional elements.* For example, if you do not eat the proper amount of protein supplying the necessary amount of the essential amino acids, your body will break down some of its own protein to obtain these amino acids.

If you are a vegetarian, don't assume that you will be skinny. Whatever your type of diet, *if you eat too many Calories, you are going to gain weight* (think of the vegetarian who eats large amounts of fatty foods such as peanut butter, coupled with large amounts of carbohydrates such as white bread, pasta, potatoes and rice, and fast foods). I'm not trying to pick on vegetarians. Most are motivated to watch what they eat and have a reasonably balanced diet. If you choose to be a vegetarian, that's fine; just be very motivated to eat well. Don't choose to be a vegetarian thinking that you will more easily lose weight.

Changing your diet and maintaining it do not have to be stressful, but **YOU DO HAVE TO PUT CONSCIOUS EFFORT** into selecting good food. You will have to make these choices **THE REST OF YOUR LIFE.** They cannot be made once and then forgotten. *You already have to make conscious food choices every day.* The only difference is that **YOU WILL BE SELECTING GOOD FOOD INSTEAD OF RANDOM OR BAD FOOD**. Once you have chosen good foods and used them for a while, **THEY BECOME A HABIT** and will be much easier to select and harder to deviate from.

Accountability

As you start to implement dietary changes, *no one is going to be looking over your shoulder* to make sure you are doing the right thing. It is *totally up to you* to monitor yourself and your progress. You will put out extra effort when you are accountable to someone else, such as your boss at work, a friend, or someone you may not know very well. However, when you make commitments to yourself, it is very easy to not be accountable for keeping them. Even if it is a reasonable commitment, you may excuse yourself for slipping on it or not completing it. Many people make New Year's resolutions that they do not keep for a variety of reasons. Part of this is usually because the commitment they make is very unrealistic and unachievable the way it was envisioned. No one is there to ask you why you are failing to keep your commitment. You do not have to feel guilty or embarrassed.

When you engage in making dietary changes the way I am proposing, you will not be accountable to anyone but yourself. You are not making any commitments except to work on **MAKING YOUR DIET HEALTHY AND LEARNING TO EAT APPROPRIATELY.** Making these changes may take months or years to get to where you want to be nutritionally and physically. There are no time commitments for achieving a healthy diet or desired weight. You will just work at a pace that is comfortable to you. Even if you are someone who has difficulty accomplishing goals that you set for yourself, **YOU WILL FIND WHAT I AM PROPOSING IS EASILY ACHIEVABLE**.

Medical Problems

There are disease states that make it difficult to lose weight (not impossible). Probably the most common medical problem is having low-thyroid hormones (hypothyroidism). Some of the symptoms of this condition are weight gain (due to reduced metabolism), very dry skin, severe hair loss, including the eyebrows, feeling cold when no one else does, hoarse or raspy voice, constipation, severe fatigue, trouble remembering things, or feeling depressed. Most thyroid problems are easy to test for and treat with replacement hormone. There are other examples of disease states and conditions that can affect metabolism. However, in **ALL** these various situations, **THE WEIGHT GAIN IS ASSOCIATED WITH EATING INAPPROPRIATELY FOR YOUR NEEDS**.

Since the intent of this book is to help you lose weight and be healthy and not be a medical text, I will leave it to you to search out more examples from medical literature. Let it suffice to know that **REGARDLESS** of your physical state, you **CAN** lose weight by eating properly for your current condition. There are **NO** excuses for not losing weight! The only way you will not lose weight is eating improperly, refusing to admit that you don't eat properly, or not being willing to try to change your eating habits. If you think you may have a medical condition affecting your weight, get evaluated by a physician.

Food Sources

One thing that I find lacking in the weight-loss literature is information showing you how to establish the healthiest diet possible on a budget you can afford. Diet programs may use certain foods that may not be affordable to you such as all organic foods. Besides being excessively expensive, *the organic cliché becomes twisted to include most foods that are widely available anyway.*

From time to time, you will hear about large producers using farming techniques that encourage rapid growth or some other aspect to increase production. This may leave the food source lacking in nutrition. A fortunate side effect of this process is that the food has little taste and is obviously different from the food you normally consume. When you encounter such food sources, simply do not use them any more than necessary. By avoiding them, reduced sales will discourage this type of production, but if it doesn't, you still do not have to use this particular food source. There are plenty of other sources of better food.

A good example of this is tomatoes. When I have encountered tomatoes from producers using growth-stimulating techniques, they are usually full of water and have little taste. I simply avoid them. Many techniques are being investigated to keep up with the increasing demand for food, and some of them are going to result in inferior products. So expect to see these types of food sources come and go as farmers work on increasing their production. The advances that produce good, nutritious food will prevail.

Another example is the use of pink meat filler to add bulk to ground meat. Nobody really noticed the use of this product until someone finally blew the whistle. It's not really harmful but allows the meat producers to utilize more of the animal. If you care about its inclusion, just ask the butcher where you purchase your meat, or don't purchase ground meat.

With current regulations and monitoring in place by the FDA, any type of chemical or process that is considered in food production is carefully evaluated. Therefore, it is unlikely that there is any significant amount of any harmful drug or chemical in our food. If there are any possible sources that might be missed, such as from overseas producers, eating from a wider variety of that food type will minimize your exposure to any potentially harmful chemicals. It is impossible to grow enough food for our population without using commercial fertilizers and pesticides. Don't let these things be an issue for getting your diet started while trying to eat as healthily as possible.

THE FRESH AND MINIMALLY PROCESSED FOOD AVAILABLE IN YOUR GROCERY STORE WILL PROVIDE YOU WITH THE NUTRITION YOU NEED. You don't need to worry about trying to buy special food, take supplements, or use any other dietary aids. **IF YOU DON'T LEARN TO EAT THE BEST YOU CAN AND KEEP YOUR WEIGHT AT A HEALTHY VALUE, NOTHING ELSE IS GOING TO MAKE A SIGNIFICANT DIFFERENCE ANYWAY.**

Calories and Nutrition

Most food products have the caloric content printed on the label. This may be a bad sign all by itself because it could mean that you are eating processed food or junk food. It does provide a quick reference for the amount of Calories you are about to consume. The food pyramids previously discussed will help you decide how to proportion your intake from each food group, but *they will not help you choose healthy food or portion size.*

The health benefit from your food depends on how much it is processed and the number of Calories per volume. Potato chips are an example of a highly processed food, high in Calories and low in nutrition. An important nutritional part, the skin, has been removed in most products, leaving the highest-caloric content, the meat of the potato. This part is then sliced and fried in very hot oil that destroys most of the remaining nutritional components and adds a significant amount of Calories from the oil. The oil is probably partially hydrogenated, which takes away nutritional value from it. Tasty spices are then added with a generous amount of salt. Now what are you left with? A slice of carbohydrate low in nutritional value to begin with and now reduced in nutrition by processing it with the generous addition of unhealthy, partially hydrogenated oil, in addition to a generous amount of salt. Now if this isn't bad enough, you do not get a feeling of fullness when you eat the chips; therefore, you can consume large quantities. Also, when you compare the Calories per volume compared to something healthy such as an apple, it is astounding how many Calories you consume for essentially a **DEFICIENCY** of nutrition. You can easily carry out this kind of analysis for numerous other foods.

Knowing detailed information about the nutritional content of food **WILL NOT** help you change your diet. Also, it **WILL NOT** help you be more nutritionally fit. The more scientific you try to make this process, the more confusing it becomes. **IF YOU EAT AS MUCH UNPROCESSED FOOD AS POSSIBLE FROM ALL THE FOOD GROUPS, YOU WILL MAXIMIZE YOUR NUTRITION.** Watching your weight will tell you if you are eating the appropriate number of Calories.

Recipes

Depending on the ingredients, recipes can make low-Calorie, nutritious dishes to very high-Calorie, low-nutrition dishes. To select a healthy recipe or modify one to be healthy, **JUST APPLY THE PRINCIPLES TO THE INGREDIENTS OF THE RECIPES AS YOU WOULD FOR ANY OTHER SINGLE FOOD ITEM.** (When you prepare a recipe from fresh and minimally processed components, you **DO NOT** have to consider cooking that recipe as processing of that food. Although cooking is processing, it is unavoidable to prepare many nutritious, low-Calorie foods.) You are already aware that foods containing a lot of white flour and/or plain sugar are high Calorie and low nutrition, and I have already pointed out the major categories. Other foods in this category are those with a lot of fat content such as breaded, fried, or deep-fat fried foods. Many recipes use items from these categories as ingredients such as pastas. Other ingredients like rice, beans, and corn can make nutritious meals that may be higher Calorie than you want or need.

When you are making your own entrée, you can control what goes into it. Therefore, it is easy to avoid or modify recipes using a lot of white flour, sugar, unhealthy oils, large amounts of fat, etc. However, when you eat at a restaurant or fast-food location, you don't have this opportunity. Therefore, it will be more difficult to determine how nutritious the items will be. The good news is that it is *very easy to estimate the number of Calories and how nutritious those menu options are.*

Single food items such as vegetables, fruits, proteins, etc., are usually quite obvious. French fries are bad; baked potatoes are good (depending on what you put on them). Broiled lean meat is good; chicken fried steak is bad. Fresh fruit is good; preserved fruit with added sugar is bad.

Other menu options made from a combination of ingredients are also usually obvious as to their nutritional quality and caloric content. When you look at the item, you can generally tell what it is comprised of. Just use the information that I have already provided you to estimate the nutritional quality and caloric content. Things that use pasta, gravy (or some other sauce made using starch or sugar), bread fillers (such as stuffing), breading, fried or deep-fried, desserts, etc., all fall into the category of high Calorie, low nutrition. Options made from fresh vegetables, whole grains, and lean meats can be very nutritious and low Calorie. There are numerous ways to prepare nutritious, tasty, low-Calorie recipes.

WITH VERY LITTLE PRACTICE, you will be able to look at a menu item and determine if it has too many carbohydrates, has too much fat, is a good nutritional choice, but has too many Calories, so you may only eat a portion of the item. Also, you are not going to make abrupt changes to your diet. Therefore, **YOU HAVE PLENTY OF TIME** to figure out healthy menu items and recipes while you are learning to eliminate high-Calorie foods from your diet and incorporating nutritious, low-Calorie foods.

Finding Nutrition Information

I am not going to talk very much about the actual caloric content or nutritional components of food, only the information you need to know to eat healthily. If you feel the need to know more detail, you can look it up in a book or on the Internet. There are plenty of good nutrition books and Internet sites available, and I don't need to repeat the information. If you use unsubstantiated sources, such as the Internet, be careful and verify their data with more than one source. People don't usually try to skew nutritional information, but they just may have a plan out there for you to embrace. Remember, if someone has an Internet site, they did not create it so they could provide you with free information. They undoubtedly have some agenda for making money from their site.

If you would rather use a book to reference this data, do the same thing. Review the contents to be sure it provides the information that you want before purchasing the book. Be careful to not get lured away from your real goal of learning how to eat well. Just ignore all the other information; otherwise, you will get bogged down in what they are promoting.

This information comes in a variety of formats with widely varying content. Many so-called nutrition books or websites are really natural-medicine resources promoting the use of their concoction of herbs. **YOU WILL NEVER NEED TO USE THIS TYPE OF INFORMATION.**

Probably the biggest reason you are reading this book is to lose weight. If you need to look up any information, it will be finding the caloric content of different types of food. For now, you should be satisfied knowing in general what foods have more Calories, and I have already reviewed them. **SINCE YOU SHOULD NOT COUNT CALORIES, YOU DON'T NEED SPECIFICS.** When you get more experience with food choices, you will be able to make a good estimate of the caloric content without looking up any information.

Conscious Effort with Small Changes

When you are making changes to any habit, the stress experienced while making that change is going to be the limiting factor in being successful. In many situations, you can minimize that stress by making small changes in the habit. **FORTUNATELY, LEARNING TO EAT HEALTHILY AND APPROPRIATELY IS ONE OF THOSE THINGS.** Therefore, when making dietary changes, you can **MAKE NEARLY IMPERCEPTIBLE SMALL CHANGES**. Although the **CHANGES YOU WILL BE MAKING ARE SMALL**, you do have to **THINK ABOUT THEM**. They are not going to happen by themselves. Over time, these **SMALL CHANGES BECOME LARGE CHANGES**. Just like an hourglass, you have to transform your bad habits (sand at the top of the hourglass) into good habits (sand at the bottom of the hourglass). This happens not all at once but a few grains at a time. Eventually, all the sand is at the bottom, and you have achieved your goal. To maintain your goal, don't turn the hourglass over. In other words, don't let yourself slip back into your old habits. However, if you do (and you will at various times), start where you are and resume making the necessary changes to continue on your path to desired weight and good health.

One of the most important things to get firmly ingrained in your mind is that **THE CHANGES YOU WILL BE MAKING ARE GRADUALLY IMPLEMENTED INTO YOUR LIFESTYLE**. There are no sudden changes to your eating habits or the foods you eat. This allows you to form **NEW EATING HABITS** that will enable you to control your weight while being as nutritionally fit as possible **EATING FOODS YOU LIKE.** Remember, these are **LIFELONG CHANGES,** not just temporary attempts at accomplishing weight loss as rapidly as possible without concern for long-term maintainability and overall health.

Just think for a minute about your favorite food or dessert. If I say that starting right now, you could no longer eat it, think about how much you would be stressed. If you don't feel the stress now, just tell yourself that you can no longer have this food item. Every time you encounter it, you have to avoid eating it regardless of the situation. Over time, you will experience the kind of stress I am talking about, and you will eat the food item. It is this stress that causes you to fail in virtually all diet plans (or in making any radical life change). **LARGE CHANGES** bring about **BIG ANXIETY,** which results in turning away from any plan. The changes that you make are going to be **SLOW AND METHODICAL.** Make them tolerable as they are going to be lifelong changes.

Now, if I say you can still have your favorite food or dessert but you just have to eat a little bit less, you would probably accept this as being okay. I don't specify how much you have to cut out, just that you have to reduce your portion a little bit. You decide how much *a little bit* means as the change you are making has to be tolerable. It may be a little change, or it could be a large change–you decide. Now every time you encounter this food item, you can still eat it, but just a little less.

As an example, you may be the person who eats a bowl of ice cream as you watch the evening news. Rather than stopping this ritual abruptly, you could just eat a little less ice cream. You decide how much *less* is tolerable and how often you will reduce the amount. Over time (several weeks to months), you will find yourself eating a very small portion, and at some point, you will start skipping the ice cream. This would be a good time to stop eating it without causing excessive stress, which will result in returning to eating your ice cream.

You will be eliminating or significantly reducing the amount of poor food choices that you eat, and adding good food choices to your diet. These will be worked in a little bit at a time, just as the bad food choices will be eliminated a little bit at a time. **YOU HAVE TO THINK ABOUT WHAT YOU ARE DOING AND MAKE CONSCIOUS DECISIONS.**

Also *remember that you are eating to be healthy, not just to lose weight.* You can easily control your weight by eating nutritionally poor food, which will result in poor nutritional health. That is why the emphasis on nutrition and not just eating less. If you feel like you have a medical condition that may make it difficult to lose weight, get checked out by your doctor. Just remember that *they may make some inappropriate recommendations*, trying to be helpful. Also **NEVER LOSE SIGHT OF THE FACT** that there is **NOTHING** *that can prevent you from losing weight.*

Postponement

There will be situations where you will not be able to make small changes in your eating habits. In these situations, a very powerful technique you may need to use is **POSTPONEMENT**. This is learning to *postpone* eating your favorite food or snack item rather than *denying* yourself. Denial can cause such great anxiety that it will be impossible for you to make these necessary dietary changes. Postponement may be the key to help you avoid some of this anxiety. *I want to make it very clear that this is a* **REAL, PURPOSEFUL CONCEPT,** *not some fleeting thought.* For most people, making any change in their lifestyle can be very stressful. Therefore, having a method to negotiate this stressful time is invaluable.

I previously pointed out some examples of postponement such as attending an event or being on vacation or many other similar situations where the potential anxiety is masked. This was a **SUBCONSCIOUS POSTPONEMENT**. You did not have to think about engaging in your ritual because it was masked by the event. What you need to use is **CONSCIOUS POSTPONEMENT,** where you purposely postpone engaging in your ritual.

For example, if you like to eat a particular candy bar at your morning break, you may experience significant anxiety if you are not allowed to have it. However, if you just put off eating part of the candy bar until later, the anxiety of denial will be alleviated or at least significantly reduced. At first, you may just eat half the candy bar and postpone eating the rest until lunch. At lunch, you usually eat something else, so you may postpone eating the other half until your afternoon break or not eat it until the next day.

As you exercise this principle of postponement rather than denial, the level of anxiety that you experience from not eating a particular food item at a particular time is minimized. The amount you eat decreases as you continue to use postponement until you can go without that item altogether. In the example above, you may have started by postponing eating half the candy bar. Soon, and you define *soon*, you will be able to postpone eating any of the candy bar. Eventually, you should avoid snacking on anything during your break. Again, how fast this occurs is up to you. It has to be tolerable, so do it at a pace that is comfortable (but not too comfortable, or you will never get there).

PREPARE TO START YOUR DIET PLAN

Now you know that **CONTROLLING THE STRESS** from changing your eating habits is what you have to do to achieve your desired weight. **CHANGING WHAT YOU EAT** is necessary to be healthy. *To successfully manage the stress* from making these changes, you are now aware that you need to *make purposeful small changes*. This will keep the stress to a manageable amount while you form new habits that will be maintained for the rest of your life.

It is important to recognize foods that provide your most useless Calories. These are the ones you will work on eliminating first. Also, you need to recognize where your diet is lacking in nutritious foods so that you can start incorporating them. You don't need specific nutrition information. As you will discover, the generalities I have provided will be quite adequate in virtually all cases.

Analyze Your Eating Habits

One of the first things you need to do is analyze your current eating habits. Do you like to snack? Do you like high-Calorie foods such as pasta, ice cream, cake, or other carbohydrate-rich foods? Are you more of a meat and potatoes person? If you feel like you already eat small meals but still cannot lose weight, get a notebook and keep track of everything you put in your mouth, except for Calorie-free foods such as water. Tally up the

Calories, and you will be surprised at how many you eat. *Most people don't realize that much of their diet is actually high Calorie and find that they snack more than they are willing to admit.* If you discover that your Calories are not excessive, then you just have to eat less or make better food choices.

For example, as you start evaluating your diet, you start with breakfast. Since you go to work early, you don't have time to eat. Therefore, you grab a breakfast bar and get an espresso on your way. On days off, you sleep in. When you wake, your breakfast consists of a muffin and coffee. Some days, you will have pancakes or cold cereal. At work, lunch usually consists of some hot dish with french fries and a beverage from the cafeteria. On days off, lunch is usually a meal with fries from your favorite fast-food restaurant. Most nights, dinner is comprised of pasta dishes with bread and, occasionally, a lettuce salad or other vegetable. Other dinner menus involve fried meat and potatoes or biscuits and gravy, etc. *Write all these items down individually or in menus.* You might sort them by the category to which they belong on the five-group food pyramid. This information will be used later. *Be sure to include anything that you eat for snacks.*

Don't worry if you don't recognize all the nutritionally poor or high-Calorie foods that you eat. At first, you might think it is difficult to do. However, I have already given you the information you need to make the distinction between good and bad food choices. After using this information for a while, you will discover that it is very easy to distinguish high-Calorie, low-nutrition food from nutritious, low-Calorie food without knowing any details about the food item.

Try to compare your diet to a healthy one. You are only going to use these diets as a comparison. If they are not perfect, it doesn't matter as you will not be eating from them anyway. Look at the menus you find and compare them to yours. *Note the amount and type of food they suggest, and see how this corresponds to what you are eating.* This will give you an idea of how much you will need to change your diet.

Be careful not to use menus from a diet or supplement program. They are designed to provide you with reduced Calories, not to have healthy, well-balanced diets. It may be difficult to find menus that will provide good examples. When you look up diets and menus, since you don't know what a truly healthy diet looks like, you won't know if they are showing you one or not. *One exception may be the diabetic diets.* They are often the most reliable for getting reasonable information.

Diabetic diet information is widely available in print or on the Internet, but actual menus are more difficult to find. The American Diabetic Association (ADA) website has some examples. Just follow the prompts on their site for *recipes* and look under *One-Day Meal Plan* (their site may change by the time you read this). Bear in mind that these are also not perfect diets and may contain processed foods that are not the best nutritional choices.

For example, an ADA diet may suggest eating peanut butter. Most peanut butters are made from partially hydrogenated vegetable oils with some added peanuts for flavor. You should now be able to recognize that this is not a great food choice. If you want to eat peanut butter, choose a brand that uses peanuts as the only ingredient. Unprocessed foods do not present this dilemma; what you see is what you get.

Evolving Your Diet

Remember that you are **NOT** going to switch from your current diet to a nutritious, healthy diet. Rather, you are going to evolve to it (at this point, you don't even know what that diet will be). For example, you may use diabetic menus as a reference. You should not try to change your diet to mimic these menus, and in fact, you will probably not eat anything like them. They will merely provide you with examples of reasonable, nutritionally sound menus.

If you are able to find some nutritionally sound diets, examine your current diet and compare it to the healthy ones composed of unprocessed and minimally processed foods. You will need to identify the high-Calorie, low-nutrition foods that you eat so you can start to eliminate them from your diet. In a similar fashion, you need to recognize nutritious foods that you are not eating so they can be incorporated into your diet.

The main thing to concentrate on as you start to change your diet is **LEARNING TO EAT APPROPRIATELY** for your needs. As you do, you will start to lose weight, and you will feel better about yourself and the changes you are making. Over time, you will make your diet healthier as you continue to eliminate processed foods and replace them with unprocessed and minimally processed foods from *all five food groups.*

If you just concentrate on eating appropriately for your needs but do not eat healthy foods, you will achieve your weight goals but will not achieve your best nutritional health. If you successfully change your diet to a healthy diet but have not learned to eat appropriately for your needs, you will be healthier but will still have a weight problem. Therefore, I emphasize both learning to eat healthily while learning to eat appropriately. As you do both of these, you will get to your desired weight and be healthy at the same time. Remember that they don't have to occur at the same time and probably won't.

Eliminating Snacking

The difference between eating appropriately and changing other habits is that *you still have to eat.* One exception to this is snacking. **YOU DO NOT NEED TO SNACK** (diabetics snack for an entirely different purpose). **MOST PEOPLE COULD LOSE WEIGHT AND WOULD BE HEALTHIER IF THEY WOULD JUST STOP SNACKING.** This is just another habit you develop, usually as a comfort measure. This may happen at work, at home after work or while relaxing when the children are asleep or away to school, or one of many other similar situations. The worst snacking occurs when you have cookies, chips, or candies lying around the house or in your desk at work. You just grab something on your way through the kitchen or from your desk as you are working. This can happen several times a day and could result in hundreds of extra Calories.

Having anything to snack on, even if it is only rarely, will keep the snacking habit alive and make it very easy to slip back into the previous snacking habit. If you really want to quit snacking, **YOU NEED TO AVOID HAVING SNACK FOOD AROUND YOU**. Just leave it at the store. If it is not around staring you in the face and beckoning you to eat it, you will not be tempted. It may take a while before you get to the point where you can completely skip the snack. When you do, completely eliminate it by not buying the snack or producing it at home such as baking cookies or other snack-time food. *(I cannot overemphasize this point.)*

Something you may be faced with is being around people who snack as you are trying to quit. This is the same as a smoker trying to quit when other people around him or her aren't, or someone trying to quit drinking when he or she works as a bartender. When the bad habit you are trying to overcome (whatever it is) is constantly in your face, it becomes more difficult—not impossible—to overcome.

When it is not possible to be away from the snacks or foods that tempt you most, you will just have to work harder on changing that habit. For example, when people you take a break with indulge in your favorite snack, you will have to become pleased that you do not have to indulge in that snack item anymore. It may take a significant amount of time to achieve this (months to a year or more), but that is okay. At least you will be there. The best situation is to have the other people around you working on eliminating the same snacking habits so you can work on it together.

Another difficult situation is when your main snacking is at home. *Unless everyone living there is working on losing weight and improving nutritional health, you will be faced with excess snacks that you cannot leave at the store.* For example, if someone in your home likes to bake cookies, they will be there and a temptation for you. When you see the plate of cookies sitting on the counter, you will need to become disciplined enough to walk away without indulging in the cookies or other snack item. If you cannot engage the other members of your household in improving nutritional health and working on weight loss, you will have to be more motivated to control your snacking habits. This can be done using the techniques in this book, but you will be constantly faced with the choice between eating and not eating a snack item.

Don't substitute one bad habit for the same one or a worse one. For example, if you smoke, you are already on a sinking ship. Don't punch more holes in the bottom by smoking more to compensate for your snacking. If you are trying to quit smoking, don't substitute snacking for smoking.

Don't forget, these are *conscious choices* that you must constantly make. *You already make food choices for snacks and meals, so you are not adding something you don't already do.* The choices you will now be making are *conscious, healthy choices, not conscious, random, unhealthy choices.* Once you make healthy choices a habit, making them will be much easier.

Success in Achieving Your Goal

If you really want to be successful at eating healthily and appropriately, you need to learn how to accomplish it in a manner that does not cause undue stress, anxiety, frustration, and ups and downs with ultimate failure. With the information contained in this book, you are aware that you need to make **SLOW, PURPOSEFUL CHANGES** to your diet that are **PERMANENT** and occur over weeks to months and maybe years. This will minimize the anxiety you would otherwise experience, which would cause you to abandon your new diet goal. Having abandoned your new goal, you have no place to turn except to your old habits that caused your problem in the first place. **IT IS EXTREMELY IMPORTANT TO GET THESE IDEAS FIRMLY PLANTED IN YOUR HEAD!**

You are now armed with enough knowledge about nutrition to help you recognize the shortcomings of any lose-weight-fast or eat-what-you-want diet plan. The information presented on supplements and natural medicines will allow you to recognize that they are not needed. I continuously see new advertisements popping up with the latest discovery, promising miraculous results. **YOU NOW KNOW THAT THEIR NEW DISCOVERY IS, IN REALITY, HOW TO GET MORE MONEY OUT OF YOUR WALLET INTO THEIRS.** Also, you have enough information to recognize most good food choices. It is actually quite easy to recognize them. *The difficulty is learning to select that choice over less healthy options.*

As you read into the next sections, you will notice that there are **NO SPECIFIC MENUS** mentioned. This is because **THERE ARE AS MANY BALANCED, HEALTHY DIETS AS THERE ARE INDIVIDUALS.** Everyone has his or her own taste in food. If I try to outline specific menus, I would be presenting a diet plan that would be similar to other diet plans (i.e., I tell you what to eat). You would also try to switch to these menus immediately without going through any evolution. The menus would probably not correspond to your taste in food and would make it more difficult to implement the necessary changes. This would defeat the intent of this book. There are many ways to eat healthily and appropriately for your needs, and it is impossible to outline a significant portion of them. **YOU NEED TO LEARN HOW TO SELECT HEALTHY FOODS THAT YOU LIKE AND EAT THEM APPROPRIATELY FOR YOUR NEEDS.** Again, there are many ways to accomplish this.

The next section will go through an example of how to use this knowledge to help you get started. *You will just keep implementing changes slowly until you have arrived at your goal (weeks to years), and then you will continue with your new diet plan, making improvements and healthy changes along the way, for the* ***REST OF YOUR LIFE.*** *Remember, you set the pace with which these changes are made. Make the changes tolerable but deliberate so that you will eventually reach your goal.*

STARTING THE EVOLUTION

Now it is time to implement a plan for changing your diet. At this point, you have been given all the information you will need to successfully change your eating habits in a nonstressful way so that you will be healthier and achieve the weight you would like to maintain for the remainder of your life. *The barrage of useless information and programs that are being thrown at you should no longer be a stumbling block or entice you to engage in useless pursuits.*

You may be wondering why I have been talking about diet but have said very little about exercise. Diet and exercise are important components of your health, but *nutrition needs to come first.* I'm going to bring this up now and will talk about it again later and in the section on exercise. This is a **VERY IMPORTANT** point to understand clearly. **DO NOT,** *in any way, shape, or form, use exercise as part of your diet program.* I know this contradicts everything you have been taught about weight loss (except for the programs that promise that you will lose weight by doing nothing while using their product). *You can easily eat more Calories than you can burn off with exercise.* Exercise is for cardiovascular and musculoskeletal health, not weight loss. **WEIGHT LOSS IS ACHIEVED AT THE DINNER TABLE, NOT IN THE GYM.** Now if you work out, it *may* help you lose weight a little faster, and if it does, you should eat a little more so you don't lose weight too fast. Just remember to cut back on your Calories if you cannot work out for some reason. I only mention this now because I know some of you are going to try to use exercise as part of your weight-loss plan. It is a self-defeating plan that leads to much frustration. Only concentrate on what you eat for now.

Address Snacking First

If you eat any snacks, you should *work on reducing them first.* Diabetics snack because they need to reduce their mealtime carbohydrate load. Therefore, they spread out the carbohydrates by consuming some of them in a snack. You will not need to do this. Whatever your snacking habits, *be honest with yourself.* If it is hard for you to visualize them or you didn't separate them from your mealtime foods when you analyzed your diet previously, get a small notebook. As you eat anything other than during a regular meal, write down the foods and the time you ate them. Look up the number of Calories and add them together. You may be surprised at how many extra Calories this can provide. Now that you have identified your snacking habits, you need to start implementing a plan to stop them.

The next thing you need to do is identify your highest-Calorie snack. When you were comparing your diet to a balanced, nutritious diet, you should have started to investigate the foods that are high Calorie with low nutrition. As I have stated, this is very easy to do, with very little practice using the information I have provided. This might be a candy bar, a pop, a bagel, chips, cookies, etc. If you are unsure what your highest-Calorie snacks are, use the product labels to find the number of Calories. When the caloric content (don't worry about the number of carbohydrates, fats, etc., just the Calories) is not on the packaging, look for a similar product and use the information from its packaging. You may need to look up the food product (or something similar) on the Internet to get the caloric information. Again, do not pay attention to the other information on the websites; just get the caloric information.

Concentrate on reducing this snack first. Do this by cutting back on the amount **(YOU DECIDE THE AMOUNT)** of the snack. Over time **(and YOU DECIDE THE TIME FRAME),** you keep reducing the amount of the snack item until, at some point, you eliminate it altogether. Remember the discussion on postponement? Now may be the time to use it.

For example, when you come home from work, you like to grab a bag of your favorite chips and sit down to watch television. This is where you decide to start. Usually, you eat half a bag. To start reducing the amount, you visually try to eat a little less than half the bag. You still feel satisfied as you have almost eaten your usual amount, but conversely, you have eaten fewer Calories. **AS YOU SLOWLY CONTINUE TO REDUCE THE AMOUNT EATEN, YOU HABITUATE TO THE LESSER AMOUNT AND GET THE SAME LEVEL OF SATISFACTION THAT YOU DID PREVIOUSLY.** Over time, you will be eating much less than you ate before and feeling good about it. After a few weeks (remember, you are determining the time frame that feels comfortable to you), you notice that you have been able to reduce the amount of chips you eat to only a small handful.

Your situation may be different. Although you have been trying to reduce the amount of chips you eat, you are still eating nearly half a bag after a few weeks. It is sometimes difficult to eat just a little bit less. In these situations, it may be easier to eat a much smaller portion and postpone consuming the rest. Therefore, you start eating only a fourth of a bag and reserve the remainder of the half bag for later. As you continue to do this, **YOU HABITUATE TO EATING A MUCH SMALLER PORTION WITH THE SAME SATISFACTION THAT YOU HAD EATING THE MUCH LARGER PORTION.** In a few weeks, you notice that this has helped tremendously as you now are eating much less than one-fourth of the bag and do not consume any chips later in the evening.

In both of these scenarios, you may now be ready to stop eating the chips altogether. If it is too difficult to completely eliminate the snack, try substituting a healthy snack like carrot sticks or celery. You may not like these two vegetables, but there are a large number of low-Calorie vegetables available to choose from. Other than vegetables, there are not too many snack foods that are low-enough Calorie and nutritious enough to use as a bridge for eliminating snacking. There are many nutritious foods that you could snack on. Depending on your situation, they may provide more Calories than you will want to consume.

If you need to substitute the healthy snack, you will at least eliminate the high-caloric food from your snack time and avoid the stress of completely eliminating the snack time. You may have to reach over a plate of cookies to get a carrot, but over time, you will be able to resist the cookie for the better snack and feel very good about yourself for doing so.

Eventually, you should work toward completely eliminating the habit of snacking. *When you continue to snack even on healthy foods, it will be very easy to slip back into snacking on unhealthy or high-Calorie foods.*

NOTE THAT THERE ARE MANY WAYS TO CREATE THIS SCENARIO. Your particular approach could be slightly different from those presented, or it could be completely different. You have to decide what is right for you. The main thing to remember is that you are only **GOING TO MAKE SMALL CHANGES TO YOUR SNACKING HABITS REGARDLESS OF THE APPROACH.** Your approach could even change periodically as you discover the approach you started with is not working as well as you hoped. In the example above, that person went from trying to visually reduce the amount of the chips that they ate to using a technique of postponement. Just keep changing your approach periodically if needed to achieve the desired reduction or elimination of the snack time. Very importantly, **DO NOT** *forget that you are working on breaking a habit* and that it may take a significant amount of time to accomplish it without causing a lot of anxiety and that is okay. If you are having difficulty, *don't let yourself get lured into trying a gimmick program* to try to eliminate the snack time quicker or lose weight faster. You will eventually win if you don't give up.

If you snack several times a day, you don't have to change all your snack times at once. Pick the time when you eat the most Calories, and work on that snack time first. As that snack time is significantly reduced or eliminated, start working on another snack time. Depending on how much you snack, this may be enough to achieve the weight loss you desire. *Bear in mind that unless you are otherwise eating healthily, you will also need to work on your mealtime food choices.*

At first, you will still buy or make the snack food but just eat less. As you wean down, you will *need to stop buying or making it* in order to totally eliminate the snack food and the snack time. You will be tempted to eat some of the snack food if it is readily available. **DON'T TEMPT YOURSELF.** Just leave the snack food in the store or the ingredients in the cupboard. It may seem difficult now, but you will be able to look at your once-favorite snack food and feel within yourself that it is not worth eating. You will also feel good about leaving it in the store or not making it at home. Your snack time may be a break at work, so this time won't be eliminated. You need to learn to do something else during this break other than snacking.

Mealtime Changes

In your particular situation, you may need to work on meals before working on your snacks. It really doesn't matter which one you start with. Eventually, you will change all your meals and hopefully eliminate all your snacking. If you feel that your meals are fairly healthy, you may still need to work on making them as nutritious as possible. Whether they are nutritious or not, *you are not going to make a lot of changes all at once.*

Choose a mealtime to start changing or improving such as lunch or dinner. Pick some component of each meal that contributes the most Calories or least nutrition, and work on changing or eliminating this component. At the same time, you will start adding items you are not eating appropriately. Work on this mealtime until you have made significant improvements. For example, when you get your lunch meals significantly improved, you should start working on your dinner meals. You should probably work on the mealtime that provides the most Calories, but it may be easier to pick an evening or morning meal.

For example, when you examine your diet and compare it to a nutritious one, you discover that you really love pasta dishes. You also note that you eat few vegetables and almost no fruit. Also, you compare your diet to the food pyramids, noting that you consume little dairy and use margarine as your spread of choice. The vegetables you eat are higher in Calories, such as corn, and you only eat three or four different ones.

During your diet review, you also note that your evening meal is the larger meal of the day. This is because you have to get up early to get to work and do not have enough time to fix a proper breakfast. Due to time constraints at work, you eat a smaller lunch. So when you come home, you like to sit down to a nice, hearty meal. This is where you decide to start.

For tonight's meal, you are going to have your favorite pasta with a creamy Alfredo sauce. (The high-Calorie food that you prefer may be something else, like chicken fried steak, french fries, fried potatoes,

Southern fried chicken, rice dishes, biscuits and gravy, smothered burritos, etc.) You put your favorite meat with the pasta and have a side of garlic bread. In addition, you probably have some beverage, but consider it to be insignificant at this point. Now this may seem like a simple meal, but it is *not uncommon for people to eat from a very narrow menu.* So what should you do to fix this meal?

First, you know that you need to cut down on the total volume of the pasta. How much should you cut down? Reduce the portion by a small amount that seems comfortable to you. **DO NOT** *try to weigh or measure the volume of pasta; just get a visual of what seems acceptable.* You usually judge the amount you eat by sight, so stick to something familiar and comfortable. Also, you are used to eating a certain volume of food, so *if you decrease the amount too much, you will not feel full or satisfied.*

You may even try eating a much smaller portion and then allow yourself to have a second small portion. *Don't think that you can actually trick yourself into eating less.* Things like drinking a glass of water before a meal don't really work. You may feel full sooner, but you don't feel satisfied. Therefore, you leave the table still desiring to eat more. This could lead to going back later for more of your favorite dish or snacking on something else to fulfill the urge.

The idea is to eat a little less without feeling like you did. This is a conscious decision. You eat enough less to reduce your caloric intake a little without challenging your desire to eat the usual amount. *Therefore, at the end of the meal, you still feel satisfied but have eaten fewer Calories.*

Every time you eat the pasta, just eat a little less (an amount that feels comfortable to you). This is a process you will continue over the next few weeks to months. After reducing the amount of pasta to a small amount, you may even skip it or postpone it until another meal and substitute a healthier, lower-Calorie dish.

DO NOT add high-Calorie sauces to your menu items to make them tasty or palatable. This just defeats your attempts at eating fewer Calories. However, there are many ways to spice up your food without adding significant Calories (most spices have few, if any, Calories). The healthy diets that you reviewed may also help you pick healthier, lower-Calorie options.

You don't have to eliminate the pasta entirely; you just have to reduce the portion to be adequate for your needs. However, to avoid falling back into the pasta habit and eat healthier choices, it is probably best to eliminate the pasta entirely (or whatever other generally unhealthy, high-Calorie food you are working on reducing its consumption).

You probably do not eat pasta for every evening meal, so evaluate your other evening meals. Pick the highest-caloric food and start reducing or replacing it just like you are doing with the pasta.

REMEMBER THAT AS YOU SLOWLY REDUCE YOUR FOOD INTAKE, YOU HABITUATE TO THE LESSER AMOUNT SO THAT YOU FEEL JUST AS FULL AND SATISFIED AS YOU DID WITH THE LARGER VOLUME. THAT IS WHY THE SLOW APPROACH WORKS SO WELL. YOU ARE FORMING NEW EATING HABITS WITHOUT REALIZING YOU ARE DOING SO.

Now, since you are also trying to eat healthier, what should you do? Try adding a vegetable to the meal. Although your favorite vegetable is corn, it is high Calorie. Therefore, start trying a wider variety and use lower-Calorie ones. It's okay to still eat corn once in a while, but when you do, eat smaller portions.

Let's say that this time, you will add broccoli. Don't overindulge. Just eat a little bit to start developing a taste for different vegetables. If you seldom eat broccoli, you may not know how to best prepare it for yourself. Try it raw this time, with a little salad dressing of your choice. You don't have to eat a lot; just try a few pieces. Next time you decide to try broccoli, steam it lightly and eat it plain or with different spices. Experimenting will help you decide how you prefer to eat different foods.

EAT FROM A LARGE VARIETY OF VEGETABLES, especially from the ones that you may not like very well, such as green bean, spinach, cauliflower, broccoli, brussels sprout, okra, etc. Don't torture yourself. Just try a little bit. Try them raw with a little dressing, steamed, or prepared in some other way that makes them palatable. Also, don't defeat yourself by disguising the vegetable in some elaborate, high-Calorie sauce. Adding a salad dressing is bad enough. You are probably better off not eating a vegetable if you cannot tolerate it raw or with a small amount of salad dressing or steaming or some other simple, low-Calorie method.

At this point, you have already improved this meal a lot just by cutting back on your pasta portion and adding a single vegetable. As time goes on, keep adjusting this meal to include more vegetables and some fruits. For example, you could have a lettuce and/or spinach salad with tomato and mushrooms and maybe throw in a little corn or a few beans. *Salads are a great way to introduce vegetables that you don't like very well.* You may top off the meal with a few strawberries, a peach, an apple, or some other fruit. If you could eliminate the pasta entirely and replace it with a piece of meat (fish, chicken, or even lean beef), this would improve the meal even more. You may have been putting chicken or other meat in your pasta dish, so replacing the pasta may mean eliminating the pasta part of the dish.

Now you may be thinking, *I just replaced this pasta meal with meat (which I may have already been consuming with this meal), vegetables, fruits, a whole-wheat roll, and milk, and this is supposed to be fewer Calories than the pasta meal?* It is probably so. Pastas are high in Calories but very low in nutrition. Even if you made an even trade in Calories, you are eating more healthily. As you were cutting back on the pasta and starting to add a few other items to the meal, you were definitely eating fewer Calories. This would have helped you get into the losing-weight mode. Remember, *you are not trying to crash diet*; you are only trying to reduce your caloric intake to the point where you are going to start losing weight slowly. At the same time, you are making nutritional improvements, which may be more important to your health than losing weight.

Additionally, this is not the only meal you are changing to reduce your caloric intake. You will work on changing all your meals (and your snacks) as you learn to eat better and develop habits to help you maintain your healthy diet. Remember, this is a **SLOW, METHODICAL, LIFELONG PROCESS,** not some abrupt temporary change that you are going to stop at some point.

Don't give up if you live in a family situation where you do not have control of the food choices or you are the only one trying to be healthier at a more desirable weight. You don't have to eat a large volume of the food available. You may have limited choices of things to eat that may not be very nutritious, but you can work on portion control to achieve your weight goals. Being nutritionally fit may have to wait until you have control of the food choices. Hopefully, your example will encourage others in your family to engage in eating better, which may result in better food choices being available.

As the weeks go by, you will slowly change your diet, making it provide the appropriate number of Calories. Most importantly, you will also be improving the nutritional value of your diet, enabling you to be healthier. Do you remember comparing your diet to the healthy, balanced diets and the food pyramid discussions? This isn't some random information designed to fill up the pages of this book. *Use the food pyramid examples to see if there are food groups you are missing and if you are proportioning your food appropriately. Use the healthy-diet examples to get a feel for a balanced diet and portion size, not for menus.* **YOU WILL BE DEVELOPING YOUR OWN MENUS THAT SUIT YOUR TASTES.** Also, remember that *I do not advocate counting Calories or measuring your food.* Doing so will just add anxiety to your health plan. Importantly, do not forget that it is **YOUR WEIGHT, NOT THE PORTION SIZE**, that is telling you if you are eating appropriately for your needs. If your weight is increasing or stable while you are trying to lose weight, you just need to decrease your total caloric intake.

If you have been at this for a while (several months) and are still having difficulty losing weight, *you may need to change the combination of foods you eat.* For example, you have now developed a taste for squash and corn. After examining your current diet, you see that it comprises a significant number of your Calories. This is where you need to cut back. Reduce its volume or replace it with lower-Calorie vegetables. You may also notice that you are eating a narrow variety, so add some different, lower-Calorie vegetables.

Another example could be fruits (or any other food group). Fruits are very good nutritionally but provide a significant number of Calories. Again, examine your diet for the amount and types of fruit you eat. If you like the large bananas, try buying the smaller ones or just eat half of one. Only eat half a pear or a peach, fewer berries, or maybe only eat fruit every other day. *Remember that small changes may be all that you need to start losing weight or quit gaining weight.*

Those with Disabilities

If you are someone with a disability, you may have to limit your intake to very small meals to keep from overeating. You may be thinking that you already eat almost nothing but still cannot lose weight. That may be true to some extent, but *you can still lose weight by eating properly for your needs.* Your body needs a certain number of Calories daily to maintain your weight. By making better food choices, you may be able to reduce your Calories, eat a larger volume of food and still lose weight, or more easily maintain your desired weight.

Depending on how well you currently eat, you may improve your nutritional health as well. If you are making good food choices, there may still be more appropriate choices. For example, you may have to eat fewer vegetables from the intermediate or low-fiber group (such as corns, beans, potatoes, etc.) and eat more from the high-fiber group (such as lettuce, cabbage, carrot, celery, green bean, spinach, broccoli, cauliflower, brussels sprout, radish, and many other similar vegetables). This will allow you to eat a larger volume with fewer Calories. Eating leaner types of meat such as chicken and fish and less beef will also help with your caloric input. If you already eat from the lowest-Calorie foods, you will just have to eat less of them.

With proper or better food choices (more appropriate for your needs), you may be able to easily decrease your caloric intake by several hundred Calories daily. Just apply the principles presented here until you get your caloric intake to where it needs to be for your present condition. *Remember that your weight is what tells you that you are eating the appropriate number of Calories. Nutritional status cannot be measured except in extreme deficiency. You will be as nutritionally fit as possible if you choose food as outlined in this book.*

Snack Meals

For some people, snack time is a very important part of their diet, if not the most important. You may find that you don't have time to eat breakfast but that you have the opportunity to grab something on a break at work. Usually, these are not the most nutritious meals and are probably high Calorie. The quick breakfast snacks and other prepared foods that you buy at the store are *not worth the Calories for the minimal amount of nutrition you receive.* If you eat them, you will probably have to give up nutritionally sound food to keep your caloric input within your limits. However tasty and nutritious they may seem, *they are not worth eating.*

Depending on your caloric needs, healthy choices may also provide too many Calories. For example, you grab a banana and bagel on your way out the door. This may be a reasonably good nutritional choice, but you have now consumed a large number of Calories. The banana is mostly carbohydrate, and the bagel is all carbohydrate, and both have a relatively large number of Calories (combination is about 350 Calories). Looking up caloric information on different options, you notice that a better choice is a boiled egg and an apple. These items have a better range of nutritional components, proteins, fats, and carbohydrates and overall fewer Calories (combination is about 175 Calories). *This may seem confusing right now, but you will find that it is very easy to make these distinctions without knowing a lot about nutrition.* The most you should have to do is look up the number of Calories of various foods you are unsure about.

REVIEW OF IMPORTANT CONCEPTS

You may be saying to yourself, "After all that was said in this book, is that all the examples that you are going to give me to help me with my diet plan?" The answer is yes. **IT REALLY IS THAT EASY TO CHANGE YOUR DIET AND LEARN TO EAT APPROPRIATELY FOR YOUR NEEDS.** You now have a process that you can use to change your diet and eat healthily and maintain it for a lifetime. How you embrace and use this plan has many variations, and I could not begin to outline a small portion of them. The main thing is to use this information in a way that works for you. Only you will know what that is. However you choose to use this information, the important thing to remember is that this process occurs **SLOWLY** so that you hardly notice the changes. They result in developing good nutritional eating **HABITS** such that you can be **NUTRITIONALLY HEALTHY** at the **WEIGHT** you desire **WITHOUT** the use of diet plans, supplements, herbs, etc. You will also be able to maintain these changes forever.

As you may recall in the section titled "The Plain Facts," I stated, "There is only you, armed with sufficient knowledge and a little willpower to use that knowledge that will ultimately allow you to achieve a lean body mass and have good health for the rest of your life." **THROUGHOUT THIS BOOK, I HAVE GIVEN YOU THE KNOWLEDGE AND ENCOURAGEMENT YOU NEED TO ACHIEVE YOUR WEIGHT AND HEALTH GOALS. YOU WILL HAVE TO FIND THE WILLPOWER WITHIN YOURSELF. NO ONE CAN GIVE THAT TO YOU. NOW YOU NO LONGER NEED TO BE DECEIVED BY**

LURING ADVERTISEMENTS, ENTICING WEBSITES, OR CELEBRITY TELEVISION SHOWS. YOU KNOW WHAT YOU HAVE TO DO AND HOW TO DO IT. NOW THE REST IS UP TO YOU.

Don't Give Up

You may notice that you are not losing or stop losing weight after several weeks or months of making dietary changes. Examine the food you eat and look up the caloric content. Cut back on the amount of higher-Calorie foods. Additionally, look up the caloric content of other choices, and determine how to substitute them to reduce your total Calories but still maintain good nutritional choices. Remember that all you have to do is look for foods (from all five food groups) that are unprocessed (raw) or minimally processed to maximize your nutrition. Some nutritious foods are masked by the use of high-Calorie sauces or breading and frying them in oil. Maybe you need to eliminate some foods from your diet or eat them less frequently. Remember that some food choices, no matter how much you like them, should be completely eliminated from your diet. These include foods such as pasta, white bread, candy, soda pop, cookies, cake, ice cream, crackers, chips, and other high-Calorie, low-nutrition foods.

You may simply need to eat less of the food you are already eating. This will be an ongoing process as you learn to eat better and more appropriately. That is okay. You are not in a big hurry; you have a lot of time to learn about the caloric content of various foods. Also, you don't really need to learn the nutritional components of the various foods if you eat from the five major food groups as I have described.

If you try to control the nutritional components you eat, you will drive yourself crazy trying to assess and balance your nutrition. Besides, **NO ONE REALLY KNOWS HOW TO COMPLETELY BALANCE YOUR NUTRITIONAL NEEDS** (although there are a lot of people out there who think they can). In spite of all the knowledge that there is concerning the nutritional content of foods and the needs of your body, **NO ONE HAS OR WILL BE ABLE TO** tell you exactly what and when to eat something to maximize your nutrition. **IT IS SIMPLY TOO COMPLEX.** Also, there is no single supplement or combination of supplements that is going to maximize your nutrition. Taking in excess supplements does **NOT** improve your nutritional state and may result in throwing your system out of balance.

Remember that health cannot be measured. Therefore, eating a wide variety of unprocessed foods from the various food groups, as previously discussed, will provide you with proper nutrition. **THE ONLY THING YOU REALLY HAVE CONTROL OF IS THE AMOUNT AND TYPE OF FOOD EATEN FROM THE VARIOUS FOOD GROUPS.** Your weight will tell you if you eat the proper amount.

Never forget that **ABRUPT CHANGE IN YOUR EATING HABITS IS THE MAJOR CAUSE FOR FAILURE**. You end up not losing weight and resorting to your old eating habits. Remember that this is a *conscious effort,* not a mindless endeavor, but also remember that it does not have to be stressful. *Slow and steady* is the key. Short failures should not bring alarm but remind you that it takes a consistent small effort over a long time to succeed.

Short-term success with ultimate, long-term failure is not success. These are the diet plans that you may have been involved with or see frequently advertised. You may see immediate results, but in the long term, you end up where you started or worse. *Short-term failure with ultimate, long-term success is not failure.* This is the plan you are now engaging in. Along the way, you are going to have setbacks (some of these might even be after you achieve your desired weight). That is okay. You just restart where you are and keep going. Eventually, you will get to your goals (months to years), but once you arrive, you have won. You will now have habits that will enable you to maintain your weight and maximize your health for the rest of your life.

Conscious Decisions

I CANNOT OVEREMPHASIZE THE NEED TO CONSCIOUSLY PAY ATTENTION TO WHAT YOU ARE DOING. You need to make slow, purposeful dietary changes. Making changes too quickly will result in cravings and increased anxiety which will result in a return to the less stressful habits you are trying to eliminate. Making changes too slowly will never get you to the point you are trying to achieve. There is no right or wrong time frame to work within to achieve your goal. Just **SLOW, STEADY PROGRESS AT A PACE YOU CAN TOLERATE** is going to get you there. This process may sound stressful all by itself, but it really isn't. You will hardly notice these small changes, but you have to consciously make them. They do not occur without some thought process. Also, remember that **YOU ARE CURRENTLY MAKING THESE CONSCIOUS DECISIONS.** *Your goal now is to make better, conscious decisions and to change your old bad decisions into new good decisions.*

Menus

Remember that *I am not recommending any particular menus.* When you consider the vast variety of nutritious food, healthy ways to prepare it, and differences in tastes of individuals, it is impossible to come up with menus that would result in lifelong changes for large numbers of individuals (although many people have tried). You now have the knowledge of what nutritious food is. Therefore, you need to come up with your **OWN MENUS** that are **SATISFYING TO YOU** but, at the same time, **NUTRITIOUS**. To obtain and maintain your desired weight, you simply have to **EAT FROM YOUR NUTRITIOUS MENUS IN PROPER PORTIONS FOR YOUR NEEDS.**

Be careful when you use recipes from cooking shows and restaurants. These are designed to set the chef or restaurant apart from everyone else, not to be the most nutritious or low-Calorie. Really be careful if you pick up recipes from weight-loss TV shows or Internet sites. Their objective is to make extremely low-Calorie meals so the weight loss will occur rapidly. You are now aware that this is a really bad idea as too much hunger brings about high stress and binging. Also, these meals are usually not very nutritious as it is difficult to provide the best nutrition and extreme weight loss at the same time.

How Fast Can You Lose Weight?

Another very important point is, how fast should you lose your weight? Once you reach a caloric intake that allows you to lose about **ONE POUND PER WEEK, DO NOT** try to lose weight faster. Faster weight loss usually leaves you too hungry and prone to snacking (or binging) or eating larger meals. Remember, one pound per week equates to fifty-two pounds per year. How much weight do you need or want to lose? There are fewer people who need to lose one hundred pounds or more (although this number is continuously rising). Most people are going to reach their weight goals in a year or less, but if it takes you two or three years to get there, so what? At least you will be there. *The best part is that you have now developed habits that will allow you to maintain that weight and be healthy without doing anything differently.*

When you start weighing yourself, you will notice that your weight can fluctuate significantly. One of the reasons is, a single eight-ounce glass of water weighs half a pound. So just drinking a pint of water will change your weight by one pound. It is not unusual for your weight to go up and down by three to four pounds or more during the day from food and liquid intake or elimination. Due to this frequently changing weight, if you try to weigh yourself on a daily basis or more frequently than once a week, it will be more difficult to differentiate true weight loss from true weight gain.

Therefore, **I RECOMMEND THAT YOU ONLY WEIGH YOURSELF ONCE A WEEK**. Also try to weigh about the same time of day to diminish changes in your weight due to intake and elimination. Mornings before you eat or drink anything would probably be the best. This could be before or after going through your daily bowel habits. Pick a day and time when you think you will weigh the most. I pick Monday morning as this is most likely the day and time where I will be my heaviest. This is because I am usually a little more sedentary on the weekends, especially Sunday, than on other times of the week.

On your weekly weigh-in, you may be a little heavier or lighter than the week before for the same reasons as the daily weight fluctuations.

However, it is okay to make minor adjustments in your food intake, but make them small. Doing so will not result in undereating and risk getting too hungry and binging. Conversely, you will not overeat and regain some of the weight you have lost.

You cannot pick up a trend on a week-to-week basis. A trend will become evident over a three- to five-week interval. Your weight will go up and down over this time period, but you will see an average. This average will tell you if you are making the correct adjustments. Don't try to calculate this average; just get an idea of the trend. It is okay to write your weight down to help you remember it. If your average weight is staying the same but you are trying to lose weight, cut back just a little bit more. If you are losing weight too fast, just eat a little bit more. *When you have made the correct adjustments to your diet, you will see a steady average weight decrease of about one pound per week.*

If you weigh yourself less frequently, you may start gaining or losing weight faster than you want to between the weigh-in intervals. Once your weight gets some momentum going between the prolonged weigh-in periods, it will be harder to make the correct adjustments in your caloric intake. Although there are a lot of different opinions on how often to weigh, *just use the weekly weigh-in plan.* It will be much easier to make the correct dietary adjustments and keep or achieve your desired weight.

Making Food Choices

One of the most important things that you will need to learn is how to make good food choices. You have probably spent a lifetime making bad food choices. Now it is time to start making good food choices. This is not difficult. Throughout this book, I have given you information on what constitutes good food choices.

The main thing to consider when making food choices is to **CHOOSE FOODS THAT ARE FRESH AND MAKE SURE THAT YOU ARE EATING FROM ALL FIVE FOOD GROUPS**. Any form of processing of all food types will result in losing some of their nutritional components. Fresh foods that can be eaten raw are the best; frozen foods are next best.

Steaming is probably the least amount of processing you can do, but this usually extracts some of the nutritional components. Unless you drink the water they were steamed in, these nutrients will be lost. Of course, the heat will destroy some of the nutrients, but that is unavoidable. Canned food is less nutritious due to the high heat and/or multiple heat cycles used during processing. Also, many canned foods have lots of added sugar to help in the preservation process. Eat from recipes that use fresh components, and avoid as much white flour and sugar as possible. Also avoid breaded foods and deep-fat fried foods to reduce unneeded, low-nutrition Calories from oil they are cooked in.

Certain foods such as meat should be cooked minimally at a low temperature. This will prevent destroying the amino acids you are really trying to get from them. Certain meats such as chicken have the possibility of bacterial contamination. It is recommended to heat poultry to a certain temperature to kill the bacteria (this value changes periodically). This will, of course, destroy more amino acids but also ensure safe eating. In the big scheme of things, this is okay. You usually get much more protein in your diet than you really need. Choosing leaner meat such as chicken may be what you need rather than higher-Calorie meat like beef. There are other lean meats, such as fish, that can be eaten raw or, if you prefer, cooked very lightly.

Choose foods according to your caloric needs. If you like potatoes and you are trying to lose weight, they are not a good food choice. Conversely, if you work very hard at your job, you may need to eat potatoes to have enough energy.

Use the generalities pointed out in the section on food pyramids to help you get started. This will ensure that you are eating from all five of the major food groups. Along the way, start looking up the Calories of food you are not sure about. It won't take long before you will recognize the caloric content of virtually all foods. Knowing the number of Calories will not tell you if the food is nutritious; just the Calories that you are receiving.

Eat the different types of food in proportion to their level on the food pyramid. In the big scheme of things, food pyramids are of little worth. However, they are useful at first to help you eat the proper proportions from the different groups. They will remind you to eat more vegetables and cereal grains. They will help you to remember fruit and dairy products, especially butter. After a short time, you will remember these things and no longer need to be reminded by the pyramids.

Because there is so much variety in most food groups, it may help if you make a list of the options available in your area. Try to eat each option at least once a week. Remember that many of your food items may be combined into a single dish. Count the components of the dish as servings for that food group.

Some things are not included explicitly on most food pyramids. Nuts are an example of one of these foods. They are quite nutritious, providing a variety of nutritional components and oils, but do have a fairly large number of Calories. As you improve your diet, you may work some of these into your meals. *Just be aware that you already get their nutritional components from other food items.* On the other hand, *obtaining nutritional components from different sources ensures that you get all the available nutrients from that food group.* **DO NOT** *try to look up the nutritional components of your food so you can balance them.* **REMEMBER** *that even very well-educated nutritionists cannot do that.*

There are several other food items you will encounter as you improve your diet. Remember that these are *real food items*, such as nuts and berries, *not supplements, natural medicines, herbs, etc.* If they are being advertised to fix some function of your body, make you lose weight, cure some ailment, etc., they are supplements or natural medicines you don't need.

You will find very few, if any, new food items as you are probably already aware of nearly all real foods. There may be some tropical fruits or types of nuts and seeds that you have not heard about that could be worked into your diet. *They will merely give you another choice for obtaining these nutritional elements.* I'm emphasizing this information as *there is an enormous amount of fruit, seed, nut, etc., products that have been disguised as supplements and natural medicines.* They are advertised to provide nutritional elements that are not available from any other source. Just remember that **IF YOU ARE EATING FROM ALL THE FIVE MAJOR FOOD GROUPS, YOU WILL ALREADY BE GETTING THE NUTRITIONAL ELEMENTS CONTAINED IN THESE NEW FOOD ITEMS, SUPPLEMENTS, AND NATURAL MEDICINES.**

Servings

If you did not pick this up from the food pyramid discussion, a serving is just the amount of a food item that you put on your plate. There has been little mention of the size of the serving. Many people define a *serving* as so many ounces. They may also define it in other measurement terms. **YOUR SERVING SIZE** will vary, depending on the food item and your caloric needs.

YOU SHOULD NOT WEIGH OR MEASURE YOUR FOOD IN ANY FASHION as this just adds another level of stress to the changing your diet process. Just use a visual measurement or other technique that you are currently using and are comfortable with. Besides, the portion size doesn't matter. What does matter is that you learn to eat portions that are satisfying to you (and the portion size will change as you change your diet) but provide the proper number of Calories and better nutrition. Remember, it is your weight that tells you how proper the volume and type of food intake is, not the measurement of your food.

A Note for the Elderly

You may not be trying to lose weight, but the information in this book still pertains to you as well as everyone else. Many elderly people suffer from nutritional deficiencies and increasing health issues. This is partly brought about because of a natural loss of appetite and reduced activity. To avoid gaining weight, you reduce your intake of nutritious food. You may not eat very nutritiously, to begin with, having settled in to a diet comprised of a few of your favorite foods. Reduced nutrition, coupled with reduced activity, results in an increased loss of health, including muscle mass and strength. This combination results in a downward spiral. You continue to lose strength as you also continue to become more nutritionally deficient. This can put you at risk for physical injury as well as increased health issues.

The aging process cannot be stopped as this is programmed. However, you can significantly alter this process by maintaining a healthy diet as described in this book, coupled with exercise. The exercise needs to be as vigorous as possible to maximize your muscle mass and strength. There is a great number of people who are sitting around, waiting to die, simply due to being nutritionally deprived and physically unfit. Don't be one of these people. At least make yourself as nutritionally fit as possible and be as physically active as you can.

If you can exercise, it needs to be comprised of things that challenge you well above what is required for daily living. This will help you avoid losing functionality as you age. There is much more that could be said about this, but just be aware that nutrition and exercise will play a major role in your health and well-being throughout your entire life. **THERE IS NEVER A POINT WHERE YOU DON'T HAVE TO PAY ATTENTION TO WHAT YOU EAT AND HOW ACTIVE YOU ARE.**

SUMMARY OF KEY POINTS

Before concluding, I'm going to summarize some key points that you are going to use to implement your diet and nutrition plan. A few of these points may have been discussed several times in various places throughout the book. Those points are very important and ones that you should pay particular attention to. Other key points that may not have been discussed as thoroughly but are very important will also be reviewed. If you have forgotten why and how supplements, natural medicines, herbs, diet plans, diet medications, surgeries, and other current ways of losing weight are fallacies, go back and reread the beginning sections discussing these topics. It is important to understand clearly that there is **NO MAGICAL SOLUTION** to weight loss.

1. Review the information about food pyramids. This will help you get an idea of the amount and types of food you should eat. This is not a guide to better eating. Notice that many food pyramids contain highly processed foods representing a particular food group. This is self-defeating if you are also trying to be as nutritionally fit as possible as you work on getting to your desired weight. The food pyramids should only be used to gain some familiarity with food groups and the relative quantities (or number of servings) that you should eat from each group on a daily basis. Once you have a little familiarity, you will not need to utilize them further. The five-group food pyramid examples I provide give you the best breakdown of the various groups without causing a lot of confusion.
2. Look at some menus representing a balanced diet. Be very careful

when you look up this information as most websites and nutrition books are going to be presenting their diet plan. Their menus represent lose-weight-fast approaches, not healthy eating. It may be difficult to find balanced, healthy menus unless they come from a website like the American Diabetic Association. Even the diabetic sites can present menus that are not completely balanced meals and the healthiest they could be.

Remember that the menus you look at are not perfect but only guidelines. You are not going to switch to or even eat from these menus. They will merely give you an idea of what your diet may be similar to once you have converted your diet to a healthy diet.

3. Compare your current menus with the more ideal menus, and decide where you need to start making changes. Start with the highest-caloric foods with the poorest nutritional content. If you find that your eating habits are fairly nutritious, you may just need to work on portion control and expanding the variety of foods you eat. Also, don't forget that many good diets are compromised by poor snacking habits. Again, be honest with yourself. Pay attention to all aspects of your food intake, whether from meals or snacking, and first work on the area where the most useless Calories are being eaten.
4. Start implementing slow, methodical changes to your meals and snacking habits. Remember, this process will take weeks or months or years to implement. What's your hurry? You spent years and maybe used numerous diet plans to get to where you are today. You have the rest of your life to eat well, so take your time, and make the journey more enjoyable and achievable.

   If you are the only one in your house making these changes, you will have a more difficult situation to deal with. Just use the information that I previously gave you and do the best you can.
5. As you make changes to your meals or maybe before making meal changes, start implementing changes to your snacking habits. Snacking is the one big thing that destroys most healthy diets and contributes to worse nutritional health. For some reason, people pay particular attention to their mealtime intake but completely ignore their snacking. It is okay to change the things that you snack

on to help you get started on improving your nutrition and losing weight, but your long-term goal should be to eliminate your snacking altogether. After all, snacking is strictly a habit. It is completely unnecessary for good health and nutrition.

Also, don't trade habits to cut back on your snacking. For example, if you smoke, **DO NOT** smoke more to help reduce your snacking. This will only increase your health risks from smoking. In this situation, your excess weight and poor nutrition might actually be better than the increased smoking.

Once you have reduced a snack item to a minimal amount, **QUIT BUYING** or **MAKING** the snack item. *If you have snacks around, you will eat them.* Therefore, when you have reduced the intake of a snack item to the point where you don't really feel the need to snack on it, don't buy or make any more. *If you should occasionally feel the need to indulge in that snack item, just buy a small portion and eat it all.* You will have satisfied that craving but not left yourself open to further indulgences. These occurrences should be few.

If you live with others who like to snack on the same foods you like, it will make quitting snacking much more difficult. You will have to figure out what works in your situation to help you stay away from the snack foods. The best situation is for all of you who live together to engage in changing your snacking habits at the same time.

6. Develop recipes you like but are nutritious. You may find many recipes that are already nutritious and can be used just as they are. Other recipes can be modified to make them nutritious. If you find recipes that use a lot of sugar and white flour and you cannot eliminate a significant portion of these ingredients, you are better off not eating from that recipe.
7. **THE WORST THING YOU CAN DO IS TO GET IMPATIENT AND TRY TO IMPLEMENT THIS PROGRAM TOO QUICKLY**. Remember, you did not get fat and out of shape overnight, so you are not going to get skinny, healthy, and fit overnight. As you start to make slow, methodical changes to your eating habits, your success will encourage you to continue. Your

persistence will result in good habits. Habits are habits, whether good or bad, and breaking away from any habit can cause an anxiety that promotes returning to the habit. The new habits are beneficial to your health and well-being, not detrimental like the habit you just changed.

8. Best of all, **ONCE YOU REACH YOUR DESIRED WEIGHT GOAL, YOU DO NOT HAVE TO CHANGE ANYTHING.** You have already arrived. If you do feel tempted to eat your favorite snack or other food items, just remember one thing: **NOTHING TASTES AS GOOD AS SKINNY FEELS.**

   Your old favorite dishes are some things you don't necessarily have to completely abandon. If you have a bowl of ice cream or go out for pasta once in a while, it is not going to affect either your weight or your health. It is the continuous or daily consumption of the unhealthy, high-Calorie foods you need to avoid. When holidays roll around, you do not have to excuse yourself from eating the meal. Enjoy it and then move on. Don't embrace it and then let yourself fall back into your old routine.

9. **UNDER NO CIRCUMSTANCES SHOULD YOU EVER CONSIDER EXERCISE AS PART OF YOUR DIETING PROGRAM**. You should only consider your food intake in relation to your weight in determining how much to eat. If you exercise, good for you. Consider exercise for musculoskeletal and cardiovascular fitness, not a tool for losing weight. Unless you exercise very intensely, it will not make a significant difference in how much you can eat. This issue is discussed further in the section on exercise.

10. **IT DOESN'T MATTER HOW MANY MEALS YOU EAT IN A DAY OR WHEN YOU EAT YOUR MEALS**. All that matters is how many Calories you eat during the day and how nutritious those Calories are. If you only eat one meal a day, you may get very hungry before you eat again. You may also find that it is difficult to eat appropriately from all five of the food groups. However, if this works for you, that is fine.

    THERE IS NOTHING MAGICAL ABOUT BREAKFAST. I know that a lot of people say that breakfast is the most important meal of the day. You can find a variety of reasons stated for this, but they are all unfounded. There really is **NO VALID EVIDENCE**, scientific or otherwise, that proves it is necessary to eat breakfast to be healthy. It will be more important for those who work very hard as they will need the additional Calories. The reality is that from supper to breakfast, your body is not going into a true starvation mode. Your body will utilize energy stores from the previous day's meals, but at this point, you are far from true starvation.

Remember that **YOUR BODY HABITUATES TO EATING INTERVALS**, so you will start to get hungry as you get close to your routine eating time. This also includes snack times. If you want to change your eating times, ignore your hunger until the time you want to eat. Over time, the hunger will not occur until the new eating time. So eat when it works best for you, and eat as many or few meals as you like; this could be four to five small meals or one to two large meals or some other option. Just be sure that you are eating a well-balanced diet which may be difficult to do in a single meal, but it's possible.

11. Many people are forced to eat at restaurants, cafeterias at work, or various other locations. This includes people who travel for their work or do not want to pack and carry a lunch from home. When you find yourself in one of these situations, *just use the principles presented in this book to make your meal choices.* If you rarely eat at one of these locations, it is not going to matter if you select a poorly nutritious item or not. A rare indulgence of poor food is not going to affect your overall health or weight.

    However, if you must frequently eat at these establishments, you need to learn to make healthy choices just as if you were at home. Most eating establishments, including fast-food locations, will have something on their menu that is reasonably healthy. *You will just have to slowly change your habits in selecting foods at these locations into the healthy habits that you are otherwise learning to make.*

    They may also present you with portions that are too large for your needs. You will have to limit the amount you eat from that selection to what your current needs are. The overall effect on your health and nutrition status will be the same as the meal choices you are making at home.

EATING PROPERLY CONCLUSION

LIFE IS ALL ABOUT CHOICES. If you stop and think for a minute, you have to make many choices daily on a variety of things. You have to decide what time you need to get up and what clothes you will wear. When you get to work, you may have to decide what you will work on that day. If you have children, you will have to decide much of their day for them. If you are a teacher, you have to decide exactly what you need to teach your students and how you will present the material. There are endless examples of decisions you have to make on a daily basis. Of course, you have to decide what you are going to eat for each meal and anything you might have for snacks.

You have been given information and a method for using it that will help you achieve your desired weight and be healthy for the rest of your life. There are many ways to utilize this information, but they all have the same characteristics—that is, learning to **EAT APPROPRIATE AMOUNTS OF NUTRITIOUS FOOD FROM THE FIVE MAJOR FOOD GROUPS.**

This book has **NO HYPE, NO PRODUCTS, AND NO MAGICAL PROGRAMS, JUST REAL INFORMATION WITH NO AGENDA.** However, **YOU HAVE TO CONSCIOUSLY APPLY THIS INFORMATION.**

THIS IS A LIFELONG PURSUIT. There is no such thing as getting healthy at your desired weight and then eating whatever you want and maintaining that weight and health. Your body is constantly changing and being exposed to chemicals and other pollutants it must deal with. Therefore, you must constantly be aware of what you provide it. If you provide a constant supply of good nutrients at the proper amount, your body will function at the best it is capable of and be at the weight you want.

IF YOU READ THIS BOOK AND SAY "WOW, THAT WAS A LOT OF GREAT INFORMATION" AND THEN DON'T DO ANYTHING ABOUT IT, YOU HAVE WASTED YOUR TIME. You need to think about and start using this information. Good luck, and remember, **DON'T EVER GIVE UP!** Now don't forget to read the next section on exercising.

EXERCISING

Exercise is probably the least understood and most poorly executed part of a health program. There are many fallacies that keep getting perpetuated, like stories about Billy the Kid, Robin Hood, or King Arthur. I have to laugh every time I hear someone say, "I would like to lift weights, but I don't want to get too big." Obviously, these people have absolutely no idea what is required to get big lifting weights, let alone how to execute a successful exercise program of any kind. These are the people who believe the advertisements claiming that for only a twenty-minute workout three times a week, they can look like the well-trained athlete demonstrating the program (you should now be able to see these fallacies on your own). People are generally misinformed about their own training program regardless of the type of training they are performing. I frequently hear people say, "I train hard, but I still cannot lose weight." They certainly do not understand that they cannot use exercise to control their weight.

This section is not a primer on exercise. There are many good books that will help you learn how to exercise to accomplish any physical condition that you would like to achieve. *I will help you with techniques to develop a training routine. More importantly, I will show you how to implement your routine so that you will be successful in maintaining it for a lifetime.*

Exercise and Weight Loss

DO NOT, UNDER ANY CIRCUMSTANCES, CONSIDER EXERCISE AS PART OF YOUR WEIGHT-LOSS PROGRAM. I know that most of you have been told by your trainer, schoolteacher, friend or have seen advertisements, doctor shows, etc., that said you need to exercise to lose weight. You should realize that this is a dead-end street just from reading the previous sections. I will give you further information that will help you understand that *exercise has its own purpose, which is* **NOT** *weight loss.*

Regardless of why you are working out (just toning up or being a professional or an Olympic athlete), **YOU CAN EASILY EAT MORE THAN YOUR CALORIC EXPENDITURE DURING AND AFTER YOUR WORKOUTS**. Therefore, the only way you can lose weight is by controlling your diet. It is true that if you work out intensely, you have to eat more to maintain your weight, but you still have to control your diet to the appropriate amount. Therefore, learn to control your weight with your diet.

Use exercise for its specific health benefits of muscle toning/strengthening, bone strengthening, cardiovascular health, and what I'm going to call *physiological health.*

Health Benefits

One thing I have not talked about so far is the health benefits of exercise. I have mentioned that **EXERCISE IS NECESSARY FOR OPTIMUM HEALTH**, but I have not explained why. The immediate, obvious benefits are for muscle fitness. Most everyone is aware that when you exercise, your muscles get stronger, and you build endurance (you can work harder for longer periods of time). It is also well-known that if you lay off exercising, your strength and endurance will go away fairly quickly through a process called *atrophy*. This was well-documented many years ago in a research study.

College athletes, who were very muscular and well-conditioned, were required to stay in bed for several days without any physical activity. Physical parameters were measured before, during, and after the extended inactive period. It was amazing how much muscle mass, strength, and endurance these athletes lost during this study. This is a clear demonstration of the dynamic character of your body. *If you are carrying mass that your body does not need, it will get rid of that mass.* The unfortunate thing is, *this only pertains to muscle and bone mass, not fat.* (Numerous studies have been done on muscle atrophy. Google *college students and muscle atrophy* if you want more information on this topic.)

When your muscles and bones are challenged (such as when lifting weights, running, doing aerobics, etc.), they will grow to accommodate the additional stress placed on them. The *muscles that are being stressed increase the number of fibers in the cells* to allow the muscle to handle the increased stress. The *bones remodel themselves* to reinforce the areas where the stress is being applied. This growth and remodeling continue until the muscles and bones are strong enough to handle the stress without straining them. *They will maintain this mass as long as the stress is being applied.* Note that the *muscle increase and bone remodeling will only occur enough to handle the stress.* If the stress is increased, they will build to handle the increased stress, and if it decreases, they will reduce their mass to be sufficient to handle the reduced stress. This is why **YOU HAVE TO WORK OUT CONTINUOUSLY TO MAINTAIN YOUR STRENGTH AND ENDURANCE.**

In addition to muscle fibers and bone density increasing, the *cells have to increase their ability to produce energy and perform other cellular functions.* Therefore, they increase the cellular components that provide energy to make the muscles move, build new fibers, restructure bones, etc. **THIS IS THE PART OF YOUR METABOLISM THAT YOU HEAR ABOUT CONTINUING TO CONSUME ENERGY AFTER A WORKOUT.** Of course, this doesn't happen all at once. As the stress is applied day after day, the cellular-component increase occurs until the cell is able to handle the increased demands. **THEY WILL MAINTAIN THESE COMPONENTS AS LONG AS THE DEMAND IS PRESENT.** When the demand decreases even for short periods as little as two to three days, the cells start to reduce these components to maintain the reduced demand placed on them. You may have noticed that after returning to a workout after a short vacation, your strength has waned as well as your endurance. However, after a short time, about equivalent to the amount of time taken off, you will be back to your previous strength and endurance level. Again, *the body does not maintain excess components that it does not need.*

THE PROLONGED ENERGY CONSUMPTION AND THE LEVEL THAT IT WILL OCCUR ARE IN DIRECT RELATION TO THE AMOUNT OF ENERGY EXPENDED AND STRESS PLACED ON YOUR BODY DURING A WORKOUT. For the typical person, his or her energy expenditure is relatively minimal. Unless you are able to work out very intensely or work very hard at your job, you will not generate enough stimulation to have your metabolism increased very much or for a significant amount of time. Therefore, you will expend minimal extra energy after your workouts or after work. *Don't rely on this factor (or anything associated with exercise) to help you lose weight.* If you can work out intensely, that is good for you. If you cannot work out as intensely, don't worry about it; just work out as much as you can. *Whatever your metabolic needs are, you need to learn to eat appropriately for them.* Remember, it is your weight that tells you how appropriately you are eating for your metabolic needs.

Now you may be wondering why your body stores so much fat. This is for an entirely different purpose. Your body is designed to store energy to allow you to exist for extended periods when food is not available. In other words, it stores the excess energy consumed for times of famine. It is not programmed to limit the amount of excess storage. As long as you continue to overfeed your body, it will try to store the excess. Of course, most of us do not experience times of famine, so we just continuously store this energy.

You may now be starting to see how exercise is essential for optimum health. **WHEN YOU STRESS YOUR BODY, MUSCLES GROW, BONES STRENGTHEN, AND YOUR HEART AND CARDIOVASCULAR SYSTEMS ARE STRENGTHENED.** Your body is now functioning as it was designed to. This results in a *huge reduction in type 2 diabetes, cardiovascular disease (including those related to cholesterol), high blood pressure, and many other diseases.* Its ability to function in a multitude of ways is increased through the stimulation provided by exercise or just plain hard work. I won't try to explain in detail all the physiological benefits as they are beyond the scope of this book. In essence, **ALL FUNCTIONS OF YOUR BODY ARE IMPROVED THROUGH PHYSICAL ACTIVITY.** That is just the way it is designed. It is designed to work, not to be sedentary. The increase in the various functions of your body stimulated by this physical activity is what I call **PHYSIOLOGICAL HEALTH.** To be **PHYSIOLOGICALLY HEALTHY,** it takes **PROPER NUTRITION,** coupled with **PROPER EXERCISE.**

How much you need to exercise to take advantage of these health benefits is unknown. It definitely takes more than a light workout for twenty minutes two to three times a week, which you hear advertised. It is true that it is better to do a little exercise than no exercise, but you will not increase your physiological health significantly *unless you can work out fairly intensely.* At a **MINIMUM,** it is going to take four or more very intense workouts for at least one to one and a half hours per week or working quite hard at your job to achieve some of these benefits. The number of workout days also has to exceed the number of days without training, and the intensity of your workouts has to be enough to stress your body. The only drawback to hard work is that many people end up overworking their body such that it cannot keep up with stress from the hard work. Therefore, over time, they end up having musculoskeletal problems that may not be reversible. However, **MOST** of their problems are also due to **POOR NUTRITION** and inappropriately working their bodies.

If you are to plot health benefits versus workout intensity on a chart, it would make a bell-shaped curve. To interpret this, mild workouts yield little physiological health benefit as you are just working within the physiological capability you already have. As you increase the intensity of your workouts, the physiological benefit increases until, at some point, you achieve maximal benefit. Further increasing the workout intensity stresses your body above its ability to recuperate between workouts, and *your physiological health will start to decrease.*

Therefore, *when you exercise learn to exercise as intensely as you can.* It is unlikely that you can work out hard enough to cause a decrease in your physiological health, unless you are nutritionally unhealthy. Hopefully, you can see how nutrition, exercise, and resultant health fit together. If you cannot exercise for whatever reason, you should at least try to be as nutritionally healthy as you can.

Elderly people, in particular, should strive to work out as intensely as possible. Many of you have lost physical function to the point that you have limited mobility. Maintaining a certain amount of physical strength is essential for you to avoid falls and sometimes life-threatening consequences. When you give up some physical function, such as resorting to the use of a walker or wheelchair, you will lose more of that physical function very quickly. *If you quit stimulating muscles and bones, they will atrophy to the level just necessary to handle the stress placed on them.* For example, if you could just barely walk and so started using a walker or wheelchair, soon you will not be able to walk at all because your muscles will atrophy further after giving up some of the stimulation they were receiving. *If you cannot exercise at all for whatever reason, just remember that nutritional health is the most important part of being healthy.*

No matter how hard you work out or provide stimulation to your body, **IF IT DOES NOT HAVE THE NECESSARY NUTRITIONAL COMPONENTS, IT WILL NOT BE ABLE TO FUNCTION AT ITS BEST.** In fact, *if you stress your body without proper nutrition, the exercise may actually be detrimental, not beneficial.* It should be obvious at this point that if you use up nutritional components and don't replace them, your body cannot repair itself from the physical stress caused by the exercise. *The success of any training program is about 70 to 80 percent diet (nutrition), with the remaining part being the stimulation from stress through working or exercise.*

The New Year's Resolution

As anyone who trains regularly can attest, the gyms get very busy around the first of the year as the New Year's resolution makers hit the gym with their resolve to get fit and lose weight. These same people can also attest that about two to three weeks later, the gym will return to normal habitation. One of the best descriptions of this phenomenon is depicted in the following story that I found on the Internet. There are several versions of this story, but I pulled this copy from Dustin Maher's website: DustinMaherFitness.com. He credits Arika for sending it to him. The original author of this story is unknown, but she describes the situation very well.

A WOMAN'S WEEK AT THE GYM

Dear Diary,

For my birthday this year, I purchased a week of personal training at the local health club. Although I am still in great shape since being a high school football cheerleader 43 years ago, I decided it would be a good idea to go ahead and give it a try. I called the club and made my reservations with a personal trainer named Christo, who identified himself as a 26-year-old aerobics instructor and model for athletic clothing and swim wear. Friends seemed pleased with my enthusiasm to get started! The club encouraged me to keep a diary to chart my progress.

MONDAY:

Started my day at 6:00 a.m. Tough to get out of bed, but found it was well worth it when I arrived at the health club to find Christo waiting for me. He is something of a Greek god—with blond hair, dancing eyes, and a dazzling white smile. Woo Hoo!! Christo gave me a tour and showed me the machines. I enjoyed watching the skillful way in which he conducted his aerobics class after my workout today. Very inspiring! Christo was encouraging as I did my sit-ups, although my gut was already aching from holding it in the whole time he was around. This is going to be a FANTASTIC week!!

TUESDAY:

I drank a whole pot of coffee, but I finally made it out the door. Christo made me lie on my back and push a heavy iron bar into the air then he put weights on it! My legs were a little wobbly on the treadmill, but I made the full mile. His rewarding smile made it all worthwhile. I feel GREAT! It's a whole new life for me.

WEDNESDAY:

The only way I can brush my teeth is by laying the toothbrush on the counter and moving my mouth back and forth over it. I believe I have a hernia in both pectorals. Driving was OK as long as I didn't try to steer or stop. I parked on top of a GEO in the club parking lot. Christo was impatient with me, insisting that my screams bothered other club members. His voice is a little too perky for that early in the morning and when he scolds, he gets this nasally whine that is VERY annoying. My chest hurt when I got on the treadmill, so Christo put me on the stair monster. Why the heck would anyone invent a machine to simulate an activity rendered obsolete by elevators? Christo told me it would help me get in shape and enjoy life. He said some other crap too.

THURSDAY:

Christo was waiting for me with his vampire-like teeth exposed as his thin, cruel lips were pulled back in a full snarl. I couldn't help being a half an hour late—it took me that long to tie my shoes. He took me to work out with dumbbells. When he was not looking, I ran and hid in the restroom. He sent some skinny witch to find me. Then, as punishment, he put me on the rowing machine—which I sank.

FRIDAY:

I hate that demon Christo more than any human being has ever hated any other human being in the history of the world. Stupid, skinny, anemic, anorexic, little aerobics instructor. If there was a part of my body I could move without unbearable pain, I would beat him with it. Christo wanted me to work on my triceps. I don't have any triceps! And if you don't want dents in the floor, don't hand me the stupid barbells or anything that weighs more than a sandwich. The treadmill flung me off and I landed on a health and nutrition teacher. Why couldn't it have been someone softer, like the drama coach or the choir director?

SATURDAY:

Satan left a message on my answering machine in his grating, shrilly voice wondering why I did not show up today. Just hearing his voice made me want to smash the machine with my planner; however, I lacked the strength to even use the TV remote and ended up catching eleven straight hours of the Weather Channel.

SUNDAY:

I'm having the Church van pick me up for services today so I can go and thank GOD that this week is over. I will also pray that next year my husband will choose a gift for me that is fun—like a root canal or a hysterectomy. I still say if God had wanted me to bend over, he would have sprinkled the floor with diamonds!!!

This story, in addition to being quite entertaining, is accurate in its description of the phenomenon that occurs every year at New Year's and, in fact, all the time, but in less noticeable numbers. *It is curious how so many people can make such firm resolve to make life changes but how very few are able to carry them out.*

Dumb Luck

I noticed a phenomenon many years ago after I was able to successfully make the transition from being a smoking couch potato to eating appropriately and exercising intensely. I just happened into this by dumb luck. As I was pursuing my attempts to quit smoking, I realized about the thousandth time that I quit, the only way I would be successful would be to wean myself off the cigarettes. Therefore, the leap from smoking to stopping would be a small step but still a very difficult one. About this same time, I was getting up the courage to start an exercise program.

I had spent several months investigating working out and decided I was more interested in lifting weights than any other form of exercise such as running, tennis, or basketball. I also paid more attention to weight lifting magazines. When I first saw photographs of bodybuilders, I could not believe the pictures could be real. How could anyone really look like that? However, for myself, I just wanted to tone up and concentrate on being strong. As I pursued my plans, over several months, I weaned myself down to one or two cigarettes a day and collected a lot of information on weight training. Concurrently, I looked into nutritional information. At the point of only smoking one to two cigarettes per day, I bought a one-hundred-pound set of weights. From information that came with the weight set, I put together a simple exercise routine that could be done in my living room. About this same time, I smoked the last cigarette in my last pack and made the leap into exercising.

After about fifteen to twenty minutes of light exercise, I was ready to throw up. I felt that my smoking caused me to feel ill, and I was glad I had quit. I would shower and sit down and rest. After a short while, I would once again feel like having a cigarette. The thoughts of how I felt while exercising, coupled with the decreased intensity of the desire to smoke, obtained through weaning myself down to one or two cigarettes per day, was sufficient to keep me from lighting a cigarette. The shortness of my workouts, coupled with their lightness, helped me continue exercising.

Over several weeks, the illness I felt while exercising waned, and I actually started to feel good while exercising. I increased the length and intensity of my workouts. Along with this, I started to really hate missing my workouts and made special efforts to make sure they happened. A few months into this, I met a person who was a well-trained weight lifter and learned many good techniques from him. This kept me involved in weight lifting and intensified my efforts to improve.

Unrecognized Stress

Shortly after this time, I moved to a different city where I continued my weight training. It wasn't long before I met someone who wanted to train together. It was great to have a training partner. You encourage and help each other in improving the intensity and consistency of your workouts. We trained together until he was transferred to another city. By this time, I was dedicated to training and trained hard by myself. Over the next few years, I had several people who approached me and wanted to train together. I was happy to have a training partner, as this really does make the workouts better. The only problem was that these new partners would show up for three to four weeks, and then their participation became sporadic. Soon, they would disappear. I didn't think too much about it although it became a common theme.

Years later, I began to realize what had been happening. It wasn't that they did not want to work out together any more or moved or had schedule changes that would not allow them to train with me. The whole thing stemmed from the fact that I was in much better shape. That is one of the reasons they wanted to train together. They thought that if they trained with me, they would soon be like me. However, once we started training together, they immediately started trying to compete directly with me on weight and intensity of workouts. After a short time (three to four weeks), they could no longer tolerate the intensity of the workouts and would start to miss and finally quit training with me altogether. *This is the same phenomenon that happens to people when they start their New Year's resolution or start a new training program or anything else they are not prepared to pursue.*

This is not a new phenomenon or discovery. It is simply a **DEMONSTRATION OF A NATURAL CHARACTERISTIC OF HUMANS.** *We are all resistant to change, especially when that change is in association with an unpleasant event.* How many people do you know who complain about their work or the city where they live or some other undesirable situation but find they are unable to change it? To do so would require one or several significant life changes. The **STRESS** experienced while seeking out a new job, moving away from family, or losing associations with people or other things with which they are familiar **IS MORE THAN THEY CAN TOLERATE.** These situations cause such great **ANXIETY** that it prevents them from acting on the changes, although to do so would result in great improvements in their life.

This same anxiety also occurs in people who try to stop smoking, drinking, or taking drugs or change any other habitual characteristic. How does this fit into exercise? When people consider their current physical condition, they start to feel anxiety. They want to have that teenage figure back or that youthful physique. As they view themselves in a mirror, they are not happy with what they see, and **THE ANXIETY STARTS TO BUILD.** This process continues, sometimes ever so slowly, **UNTIL THE NEED TO ACT OCCURS.** This is when the New Year's resolutions happen or when you respond to the advertisement to join a facility at a great introductory rate or when you buy that new piece of equipment you saw advertised on television, especially since you can get it for very little initial investment.

You spring into action and join the health club or call that 800 number to get started on your new quest. My, how good you feel! Finally, after having all that anxiety for so long, you are doing something about your physical condition. That first day at the gym goes something like the story previously related. You finish that first workout exhausted and achy but resolved to continue. As time goes on, the situation starts to change. Your newfound energy and commitment to training are now met with **A NEW ANXIETY.** *This is brought on by the onslaught of pain, fatigue, physical illness, and mental stress* **FROM THE EXTREME CHANGE IN YOUR PHYSICAL WELL-BEING.** Now the enthusiasm toward your new goal is met with anxiety that suppresses your enthusiasm, and *within a short time, two to three weeks, the* **ANXIETY** *has built to the point that you can* **NO LONGER PURSUE YOUR GOAL,** and you quit going to the gym amid a variety of excuses that have no merit.

What happened to the training partners? After all, they had been training for a long time and were in reasonably good shape. They were going to the gym regularly and had reasonably good training habits. *The phenomenon is the same.* Although they had been training for a long time, it was not nearly at the level they were now expecting to perform. They experienced the same anxiety buildup that the person with the New Year's resolution experienced. It just took them a little longer to reach the "I can no longer do this" point, thus the three to four weeks that they would train before returning to their former training or whatever they did.

This, apparently, is a hard concept to understand, accept, or believe. There is something that keeps people from understanding and using it to their advantage. Once I discovered this phenomenon, I tried to explain it to the next few training partners. This seemed to have little impact on their enthusiasm, and they continued to approach our workouts with the same zeal, with the same outcome. Within a few weeks, they would quit training with me. Maybe I just had bad body odor or bad breath and was unaware. I had considered many factors that could have caused this result, and I am quite sure that it was not my body odor or bad breath that drove them away. There were a couple of successful training partners that I had to quit training with. We still kept in touch, so I know there was not an anxiety separation nor a problem with body odor or bad breath.

When I have discussed this phenomenon with people who have experienced it, they know exactly what I am talking about. For example, people who train regularly and intensely immediately recognize the principles because they have experienced them. They understand the anxiety associated with training start-up and have learned how to successfully negotiate the critical times until the anxiety turns into a driving force to keep them going to the gym.

Once you get past a critical point, this anxiety becomes **A GOOD ANXIETY** *as it encourages you to excel rather than give up. Learning how to control this anxiety is extremely important for anyone who wishes to master his or her physical fitness goals.* Also, learning how to recognize and control this type of anxiety will help with other life-changing situations.

Negotiating the Critical Time

The Anxiety Monster

When you start exercising, although you are not changing jobs or moving to a new city, you are making **A MAJOR LIFE CHANGE.** When making that New Year's resolution, you prepare yourself mentally and get up the courage to sign up at the gym. What **YOU FAIL** to do is **PREPARE YOURSELF MENTALLY** for the **PHYSICAL BASHING** that you are about to undertake. You manage to muster the courage to get through the first few workouts. However, as time goes on, the mental stress experienced from the unwelcome physical stress strips away the hope you had for a new beginning. **THE GYM NOW BECOMES YOUR ENEMY** instead of your hoped-for friend, and you find any excuse to avoid going.

After a few months or years (most people require about *two years* to recover mentally), the memory of this anxiety fades, or rationalization sets in, and you start building the courage to start again. When the courage reaches the appropriate level, you renew your gym membership or take advantage of the next big special. You start over, **ONLY TO BE MET WITH THE SAME MONSTER THAT CHASED YOU FROM THE GYM BEFORE,** and the cycle is repeated. Sadly, you are still fat and out of shape. The hope is that you will find time or get a new job or some other life change that will allow you to pursue the gym. What you don't realize is that it is not your current life situation that made you fail at the gym. **IT IS THE ANXIETY MONSTER THAT ATTACKS YOU EVERY TIME YOU ATTEMPT TO GET STARTED.** To succeed, you need to learn how to deal with the anxiety experienced at the gym.

At this point, you may have been thinking about athletes who are in poor physical shape and then take a physical and mental bashing when they start training camp. Why don't they quit? (There are even a few of these people who quit.) Although they are experiencing similar physical and mental stress, they have a major incentive to help them persist through the intense training. This might be a high salary or a prestigious position on the team. Also, they are probably not in as poor physical condition as most people are when they attempt to start an exercise program. An additional factor is that they know the training will only last for a short time before they start reaping the rewards of competing. Therefore, they can successfully negotiate the critical times to get through the training. There are always exceptions to any situation you can imagine. You will find those individuals who can be in extremely poor physical condition and start pursuing an intense training program from the beginning and tolerate the physical and mental stress involved. These people are few and far between.

Dealing with the Anxiety Monster

What I inadvertently discovered and what you need to learn is that the best way to deal with this type of anxiety is to approach it **SLOWLY.** This ensures that the level of anxiety experienced is small enough that you can handle the mental stress from the physical exertion. You need to learn to approach the gym like you would eat an elephant. Not all at once but one piece at a time. If you try to eat the whole elephant, you would soon make yourself sick and would not be able to look at the elephant without vomiting. The same thing applies to working out. If you go to the gym and **BEAT YOURSELF UP THE FIRST DAY,** you will learn to **HATE THE GYM VERY QUICKLY.** It will take a long time to lose this bad feeling when you think of working out. These feelings are **MOSTLY SUBCONSCIOUS.** You don't realize why you can't get yourself to go to the gym; you just make up any excuse to not go without knowing the real reason.

You need to **START YOUR WORKOUT ROUTINE SLOWLY AT A VERY TOLERABLE LEVEL MENTALLY AND PHYSICALLY.** As time goes on, you increase the intensity of your workouts as your ability to mentally tolerate the increased physical stress increases. **OVER TIME, YOU WILL BE ABLE TO TOLERATE VERY INTENSE WORKOUTS AND EVEN LOOK FORWARD TO THEM.** In fact, you will reach a point where missing a workout will cause you so much stress that you cannot let yourself miss a workout. Only now this stress is good for you as it will keep you working out, not keep you from working out.

Also don't forget that **YOU HAVE TO GET STARTED BEFORE ANYTHING WILL HAPPEN.** If you procrastinate getting started, you never will. You cannot say, "I will start setting up my routine next week or even tomorrow." You have to say, "I'm going to start today." It doesn't have to be much. Just start thinking about what you would like to do for exercise. Once you get started in any fashion, it will be much easier to keep working at it.

If this discussion sounds similar to the discussion in the dieting section on making changes to your dieting habits, you are correct. There really isn't any difference in the anxiety felt when making changes, whether they are dieting, exercising, getting a new job, moving to a new city, trying to stop smoking, or many other significant life changes. Many life changes cannot be done in gradual fashion, such as moving to a new city or changing jobs. Therefore, the anxiety caused by these situations has to be handled all at once. However, *the stress caused from dietary and exercise changes may be handled slowly, a little at a time, making the stress very minimal and very tolerable.* The success rate for dieting and exercise will be high if you follow the information in this book.

You are now aware of the pitfalls of getting started on an exercise program. If you are going to be successful at establishing and maintaining a long-term exercise program, **IT IS IMPERATIVE THAT YOU LEARN TO NEGOTIATE THE START-UP PERIOD.** I will show you how to set up your routine and get it started by avoiding these pitfalls. The techniques I will show you are applicable to any type of training. *Heeding my advice will enable you to use exercise as part of your health program* *for a lifetime.* The following sections will help you with techniques to establish your workout routine in a way that will allow you to avoid the anxiety monster.

First Figure Out Your Routine

There are **MANY** ways to exercise to be physically fit and achieve good physiological health. It usually requires a book to describe any physical fitness program in detail; therefore, I am not going to discuss any particular program. However, the difficulty for nearly everyone is being able to establish an exercise program. **ALMOST WITHOUT EXCEPTION, ALL FAILURES OCCUR DURING THE PERIOD OF TIME YOU ARE TRYING TO INITIATE YOUR WORKOUT ROUTINE.**

To get started, forget that New Year's (or any other) resolution you have made to get in shape. It is probably unrealistic and unobtainable the way you envisioned it anyway. *Don't be in a hurry.* Take your time developing your workout routine and getting it started. This could take eight to sixteen weeks or longer, depending on how familiar you are with the type of training you will pursue.

There are two aspects to this. First, figure out your long-term physical fitness goals. Do you want to be a long-distance runner, swimmer, bodybuilder, team basketball player? Or do you just want to be able to get off the couch and go to the refrigerator for a beer without getting winded? If you cannot think of a particular physical fitness goal, just plan on doing a general workout that will include aerobic and resistance components. Next, figure out what exercise program you need to pursue to reach your goal. Now you say, "This is all great, but I haven't the foggiest idea on how to set up a routine, what exercises I can do or should do." There are several ways to go about this.

Family Physician Help

First, **DO NOT** go to your family doctor and ask for advice. Unless that person is knowledgeable about the type of training you need, he or she will not be able to give you proper information. Additionally, if he or she does have that knowledge, he or she will not have time to properly instruct you. So in either case, you will come away from that encounter worse off than before you went to see him or her. *He or she may even give you advice that will lead you to fail* from the same phenomenon, causing most other people to fail, as discussed in the beginning of this section. His or her intentions are good, but some people are just afraid to say "I don't know" and are compelled to give you information even if it is not what you need and may not necessarily be true. However, unless you know that you are in good enough physical condition to exercise, it may be a good idea to see your primary care physician and get a physical before starting to work out.

Books and Internet

There are many good books and Internet sites addressing just about any type of physical exercise or athletic pursuit. You need to be careful when using any physical fitness information as *there are many fallacies being perpetuated concerning exercise.* This will be particularly true if you are pursuing a general workout without a specific goal in mind. Notice that when you read the information, it will probably *not tell you how to get from being a couch potato to being the type of athlete you want to be.* The exercises and activities you need to perform will be described. They will also tell you how to perform the exercises and at what level you need to perform them. This will give you some idea of what you need to do once you have achieved full workout intensity. *How to get from being a couch potato to doing this full workout will be described shortly.*

Personal Friend

You may already know some people who are successful in doing the activities you would like to pursue. They may be a good resource for figuring out what training you need to perform, but again, they are probably not a good resource to help you implement the training. Starting to work out with them could be like the people who wanted to work out with me. You could be the training partner who disappears into the night after a few inappropriately hard workouts.

Trainers

Don't forget trainers at the gym. They are very knowledgeable about working out with a variety of goals in mind. They can give you all kinds of tips on appropriate exercises, setting up routines, determining your physical condition, etc. Just be aware that **THEY MAY ALSO PROMOTE MANY OF THE FALLACIES BEING PERPETUATED.**

There are a couple of things you need to consider about trainers and gyms. For gyms and trainers alike, there are advantages and disadvantages to having a large membership at a facility. If there are not enough members, the facility cannot remain in business, or the cost of membership would be prohibitive for most people. On the other hand, if there are too many members, it would be impossible to work out at their facility. So there is a balance between cost of membership and number of members. Most facilities rely on the fact that most people who purchase memberships will not use the facility on a regular basis or not at all after a short time. They are probably not aware of the phenomenon as described in this book but are aware of the statistics on the lack of use of a facility by most members. As their need for revenue waxes and wanes, they have periodic membership specials. Members translate into revenue.

Trainers are in a similar situation, but theirs is slightly different. The more members there are, the more likely they are to have a continuous supply of clients. Most members cannot afford to hire a trainer for an extended period of time. Therefore, the trainers are more or less dependent on a steady supply of new clients. Whether or not they understand the principles presented here, it is not to their advantage to help people establish and maintain a long-term training program. If they did, the gym would fill up with people who didn't need their continued services, and there would be no room for new clients, and both the gym and the trainer would experience a loss of revenue.

Don't read more into this than what I intend. There is no effort or program in place by the gym or trainer to purposely use these principles to control the flow of members through the gym. The fact that people behave this way is well-known, and the gym and trainers must use the statistical advantage of this phenomenon to survive.

If you decide to use a trainer, there are a few things you need to be aware of. Trainers are very knowledgeable in exercise, but most have **NOT BEEN TAUGHT ABOUT THE PHENOMENON I HAVE BEEN DESCRIBING.** Therefore, they will be unlikely to help you negotiate the start-up time successfully. Remember the story related earlier about the trainer at the gym? This is exactly what may happen to you and happens to most people going to the gym with or without a trainer. I constantly see trainers working poor old clients to death. They just want to be able to move so they can go on vacation next year, but they are being trained like they are trying to become bodybuilders. Why? Consider the discussion above, and come to your own conclusion.

Trainers can give you a lot of good advice on various exercises and how to perform them appropriately. They can also help you put together the routine that is right for you. If you choose to use a trainer, make sure that you **INFORM** him or her **THAT YOU ONLY WANT HIM OR HER TO HELP YOU ESTABLISH A ROUTINE, NOT TO TRAIN YOU.** Otherwise, you may find yourself looking like you are being dragged through the wringer and will soon be quitting your efforts to exercise.

They may offer to help you with a dietary plan, but I would **DECLINE THE OFFER.** If they set you up, it will be with one of the commercial dietary plans with the probable use of supplements, etc., which you now know are poor ways to approach weight and health goals. Another feature will be to use exercise as part of your weight-loss plan. By now, you know that this is a really bad idea.

Where Will You Work Out?

Next, find a gym close to home or work that has a nice environment and the facilities you want. You may not be interested in or financially able to go to a gym, which is okay. For now, assume that you are planning to go to a gym for the sake of this discussion.

Don't go to a gym that specializes in weight lifting if you want to be a swimmer, or don't drive across town just to take advantage of their membership special. Once you have located the gym or some other facility you want to join, wait for a sign-up special. They always have periodic sign-up specials to attract revenue. You have probably spent years getting fat and out of shape. Also, you are about to embark on an activity that you will have to maintain for *the rest of your life,* so what's the hurry? If you can't wait, go ahead and spend the extra money to get started sooner. Now that you have your workout location picked out (which may be your home or some other noncommercial location) and your membership in place, you are ready to begin establishing your workout.

Put Your Routine Together

After you have figured out your exercises and established a place to work out, put your exercises in an order that works well for you. This can be done before you go to the gym or while you are at the gym. There are a lot of ways to arrange your exercises, and the arrangement will change periodically. Unless you are trying to be a competitive athlete, the order is not going to make a significant difference. If you use a trainer to help you put together a routine, you may have already completed part of this step. Again, **DON'T LET THE TRAINER PUSH YOU INTO WORKING OUT TOO INTENSELY OR PURSUING SOME DEAD-END DIET PROGRAM.**

Whatever your workout routine will be, you need to plan **AT LEAST A ONE- TO ONE-AND-A-HALF–HOUR WORKOUT THAT CAN**

BE PERFORMED AT LEAST FOUR TIMES A WEEK. This is the **MINIMUM** amount of time that you will have to spend to achieve any significant level of physical condition (tone, muscle strength with increased endurance, and strengthening of bones) and a reasonable level of physiological health (increase in various functions of your body). *Your workouts will also have to be quite intense.* If you have limitations in your ability to work out, still try to work out as long and intensely as you can.

For your resistance exercises such as lifting weights, plan on doing fifteen repetitions with each set and at least three sets of each exercise once you reach the *maximum* level of your workouts. However, *to start, only perform one or two sets with only three to five reps per set with very light weights.*

If you are primarily going to perform cardio or aerobic exercises, establish times for each exercise to only take up about two-thirds of your final workout time. Reserve the rest of your time for resistance training. *To start, only run or use the stepper, etc., for five minutes or less for each exercise.*

As you put your routine together, start trying it out. At first, you will be in horribly bad shape. That's why you started all this in the first place. **DO NOT** try to get in shape all at once. *Slow and light* is the key. At first, only spend ten to fifteen minutes at the gym. During this start-up time, figure out how much weight to use, how fast you can easily walk on the treadmill, how much resistance to use on the bicycle, etc.

Each time you go to the gym, try a few different exercises. Keep adjusting the way you perform them until you know how you will perform all the exercises in your routine. As you get in better shape, expand your workout **SLOWLY** by periodically adding a little bit of time and a few exercises to each session. This is just like changing your diet. You decide how often to increase the time and which exercises to include.

Eventually, you will have included all the exercises that you will perform into one session, including cardio and resistance. *Note that you may have to reduce the weight for your resistance exercises or reduce the time on cardio machines as you add more exercises to your workout session.* This is because the light weights used at the beginning of your shorter workout session may now feel like heavy weights or because five minutes on a stepper may feel like a half hour at the end of the longer session. As you add exercises, make sure you **CONTINUE TO LEAVE THE GYM FEELING GOOD AND NOT STRESSED EITHER PHYSICALLY OR MENTALLY.** If you do, reduce the weight and/or repetitions or difficulty of aerobic exercises until you are not stressed at the end of your workout.

As you **SLOWLY** work through your entire routine, keep making changes until you get it the way you want. You may be into this process several weeks, and if you are, that is great; you are not in too big of a hurry. Now that you are working through your entire routine, continue to do it at a slow pace with very light weights where you use them. You may have started some of your exercises doing five repetitions with ten pounds. After adding more exercises to each workout, you may have had to reduce the weight to five pounds and only do four reps to avoid being stressed. Once your routine is set, you can slowly start to increase the weight and repetitions of your resistance exercises and the time and difficulty of your aerobic exercises. Every few workouts, try to add another repetition, increase your weights a little bit, or work through your routine a little faster (this may be an almost undetectable change, but you determine how fast you will do this).

Initially, you will not take up the time allotted, one to one and a half hours. **START LIGHTLY AND SLOWLY.** Just get through your routine without feeling any stress or fatigue, and at the end, you should feel like you have not done anything. Remember that at first, you will only work out for ten to fifteen minutes. Once you have your entire routine together in one workout, it may take you thirty to forty minutes to complete your ninety-minute workout. *Remember, if you feel fatigued or stressed, back off on your routine until you get in better shape.*

Leave the gym feeling great like you are preparing to go on vacation and are excited about returning next time. This is very important to help you stay on your routine. Increasing the intensity too quickly could result in stress and anxiety, which may ultimately result in you quitting your routine. **YOU NEED TO EXERCISE THE REST OF YOUR LIFE, SO DON'T GET IN A HURRY.**

Continue to slowly increase the weight used for each exercise and the number of repetitions and to walk or run a little faster. Eventually, you will be performing all your exercises with the maximum number of repetitions per exercise at the desired weight and the desired aerobic times for running, bicycling, etc. **IT IS VERY IMPORTANT TO STAY WITHIN YOUR ALLOTTED TIME.**

It may take several weeks or months of training before you start reaching this level, but that is okay. At this level, you will not be able to make further increases in the weights or run faster or increase other aspects of your routine without increasing your workout time, number of workouts, or both. **YOU HAVE NOW REACHED YOUR MAINTENANCE LEVEL.**

If you have not reached the level of physical fitness you set out to achieve, you may need to add more time or workouts to your original plan. *Just make sure you are working out as intensely as you can during your present workout sessions.* It is unlikely that you will reach your desired fitness level using less time and fewer workouts than you originally planned. You almost always underestimate the required workout effort.

To maintain this level of physical fitness, **YOU WILL HAVE TO CONTINUE TO WORK OUT AT THIS INTENSITY.** Otherwise, you will lose musculoskeletal and physiological fitness, as previously discussed.

Something else starts happening. As you continue going to the gym and leave feeling good each day, you start looking forward to your workouts. They are not burdensome or unpleasant, although you may be very tired after performing an intense workout. When you start feeling better overall, more toned, a little loosening of the waistband (from a more appropriate diet) and, most importantly, feeling good when you leave the gym, you are making the transition between being at risk for hating to go to the gym and having it become an integral part of your life.

Now you look forward to going to the gym and, in fact, go out of your way to go. You would rather miss a good movie or dinner to make sure you can work out. What a stark contrast to the story portrayed at the beginning of this section. Now that you have reached the point where you go to the gym and work out very intensely and leave the gym feeling good, **YOU HAVE MADE THE FINAL TRANSITION FOR SUCCESS.**

The Stress Monster Successfully Negotiated

Throughout the process of establishing an exercise program, you avoided the phenomenon I have been talking about. With the slow start and gradual approach, you did not experience significant anxiety or stress. As you gradually increased your workout, your body made physiological changes without producing the mental strain that occurs when hurrying the process.

In the story at the beginning of this section, the person going to the gym experienced great anxiety and mental stress. Something that initially seemed pleasant became a horrible nightmare. Physically, except for sore muscles and some aches and pains, her body managed to get through the rigorous exercises, but the mental stress was too much, resulting in her avoidance of the gym. The gym was now associated with torture rather than a tolerable or even desirable physical experience.

To summarize this phenomenon, humans characteristically avoid unpleasant situations even though they know they are necessary for their well-being. An example would be going to the dentist or doctor. You avoid making an appointment until the unpleasantness of your problem is worse than the unpleasantness that you expect to experience at the office visit. Exercise is perceived in a similar light. Once the unpleasantness of an improperly approached workout has been experienced, the anxiety and avoidance of the unpleasant event are the same. The dentist- or doctor-visit experience may not be changeable, **BUT THE EXERCISE EXPERIENCE CAN BE CONTROLLED.**

A slow introduction to exercise, which otherwise could be unpleasant, turns it into a desirable, unpleasant experience. The physiological changes that occur happen slowly enough that the brain does not perceive them as undesirable. Once the benefits of the exercise start occurring and once you can mentally tolerate the stress, you are able to maintain and even become **ADDICTED** to the routine. Some people relate this to endorphins that are released during exercise and to the pleasure or euphoria experienced from them. Whether it has anything to do with endorphins or not, you do reach a point where the benefit from the workouts becomes very desirable, and you strive diligently to maintain the workouts to continue to reap the benefits.

Layoffs from Working Out

Now that you have reached the magical time that your workouts have become a desirable part of your life, you never have to worry about having to go through that trial again, right? **WRONG!** Undoubtedly, if you maintain your workouts long enough, you will encounter circumstances that will cause you to miss long periods of workouts. Once you do, **YOU WILL BE FACED WITH STARTING OVER AGAIN.**

HOWEVER, YOU NOW KNOW HOW TO WORK YOURSELF BACK INTO AND BE ABLE TO MAINTAIN YOUR WORKOUT ROUTINE. Whether the layoff is long (years) or short (weeks to months), you will find the phenomenon is the same. As you think about going back to the gym, the anxiety will build as you think about how difficult it is going to be to perform your routine at the level you were at when you last worked out.

Remember, you don't need to restart working out at the level you were at when you started missing workouts. In fact, you do not want to even come close to working out at that level when you restart your routine. *Just go back to the gym, doing your routine lightly as you did in the beginning, and slowly increase it as you did before until you are back at your previous level.*

I have personally experienced layoffs from weeks to months. Each time I am faced with the same anxieties, as you will be, my approach is the same as described above. As I think about performing the intense workouts I left behind, I have these same anxieties, and I remind myself that I don't have to perform at that level and make plans to resume at a much-reduced level. That encourages me to get started back. Once I get back to the gym and start doing my routine lightly, I am encouraged to continue. In a short time, I find myself back at the previous level prior to the layoff, and I once again look forward to being at the gym and working out intensely.

Getting Started—Putting It All Together

You now have all the information necessary to establish and maintain an exercise program successfully. To help you get a better understanding of setting up your routine and getting started, I'm going to review the steps involved and give you an example.

It has only been three months since you have committed to working out, and so far, you haven't lifted a finger. Congratulations! You have not been in such a big hurry that you have defeated your efforts already. Remember, you didn't get fat and nutritionally unfit in a day, and you are not going to reach your ultimate goal in a day, week, month, and maybe several years. So what? You are embarking on a **LIFELONG** adventure, so take your time.

Let's imagine that you want to run and that you have set a goal to be able to run ten miles in one stretch. First, you need to do some research on running. You may have a friend or trainer to help you put together a routine. Just remember that there are many *fallacies* being perpetuated about physical training. Many of these are being **PROMOTED BY SUPPLEMENT MANUFACTURERS.** It is **UNLIKELY** that a **TRAINER** will be able to help you avoid many of these fallacies and *might promote some of them in ignorance*. Just do the best you can and especially **AVOID USING ANY SUPPLEMENTS TO HELP YOUR WORKOUTS,** as the only supplements you or anyone else needs are good food.

During your study of training routines for runners, you discover that you need to work your upper body as well as your legs to achieve maximum running physical fitness. In addition to running for leg strength and endurance, you find that you should do some exercises such as leg presses, leg extension and curls, calf raises, etc. Working your upper body may include exercises such as bench presses, bicep curls, pull-downs, hyperextensions, and others. Your routine includes upper-body, leg, core, and running components. List the exercises that you want to perform in the order you would like to start doing them. You also decide you will perform these exercises for ninety minutes four times a week when you perform your routine at its *maximum level.*

Next, look for a facility where you can train (maybe this will be your home; it doesn't matter as long as you can perform the required exercises). You may have joined a facility to gain access to a trainer to help you establish a routine. Therefore, you may have already completed some of the following discussion. Now that you have found a facility and information on the type of physical activity that you would like to do, it is time to start putting the two together. Go to the facility you have selected, and get familiar with the equipment that fits the exercises you have chosen. This will involve learning how to perform your exercises correctly and then putting the exercises in the order you will perform them.

When you are figuring out how to use the machines or free weights or whatever you will use for each exercise, make sure you learn how to perform the exercise correctly without cheating. *Cheating involves performing maneuvers that make the exercise easier to do*; therefore, you do not get the full benefit from the exercise.

At first, you will perform the exercises at **MINIMUM LEVELS** that **DO NOT CHALLENGE** you at all. For example, if you are including bench presses with your upper-body routine, start with a few repetitions, say five, and then only perform one or two sets using really light weights, maybe five pounds. Only perform your aerobic exercises for a short time, such as three minutes, at a very easy pace.

Use the time spent learning now to perform your exercises as your workout. After you know how to perform all your exercises, start performing a few of them with each workout. Initially, you should only spend about ten to fifteen minutes per workout. This probably isn't enough time to perform all your exercises; therefore, perform different ones at each workout until you have performed all your exercises. Keep slowly adding exercises to each workout. Eventually, you will be performing all of them together in a single workout.

The initial weight may seem ridiculously light for a particular exercise when performed by itself, and the aerobic exercises may seem ridiculously easy. *However, you may find that the very light weight or the easy aerobic exercise used in the beginning of your routine may now be quite heavy or difficult at the end, and you may be very fatigued.* You may even have to lighten the weight more or reduce the time on each exercise as you add exercises to your workout. Otherwise, you may feel too stressed at the end.

You are not trying to compete with anyone but yourself. Remember that over time, as you get in better physical condition, you will be able to add more and more weight and increase the number of reps and sets and increase the aerobic times until you reach the desired number of sets and time for each exercise. Even though your initial workouts may seem ridiculously light, you are still burning energy and fatiguing your muscles.

Allow minimum rest between resistance-exercise sets, or perform the exercises in pairs. When you perform exercises in pairs, keep the exercises in the same muscle group, and perform them with minimum rest between sets. For example, you may use bench presses and flies as a pair. Do a set of bench presses, and then immediately do the flies. Rest as little as you can before doing your next series of bench presses and flies. Doing exercises in pairs requires less rest between sets than if you perform the same exercise for two or more sets in a row. This is a technique for keeping the intensity of your routine higher. It is also an advanced technique. I only mention this now because few people actually work out in this fashion, although it greatly enhances the effectiveness of your workouts.

Another technique for increasing the intensity of your workouts is to perform your exercises one after another in a series. Once you get through all your exercises, repeat the series until you have completed the number of sets you are planning to perform. This is usually two or three sets, but you may be using another plan. The problem with this method is that your muscles get too much rest between sets, and therefore, there is not as much stress and stimulation to make them strengthen and grow. If you don't care about getting the maximum benefit from your workouts, this technique is fine.

You will probably find that your routine can be done in twenty minutes, plus the sixty minutes you plan to run. Only at this point, you are only walking slowly for five to ten minutes for the running portion of your routine. So now your routine can be done in twenty-five to thirty minutes (remember that it has taken you several weeks to get to this point). This is great. Go through your routine. At the end, you should feel like you haven't done anything. Perfect. If you feel stressed at all, decrease your routine until it can be accomplished with very little effort. **LEAVE THE GYM FEELING GOOD AND LOOKING FORWARD TO COMING BACK AGAIN.** If you do this, you are on your way to successful exercising.

As time goes on, you will keep increasing the intensity of your workouts by increasing the weight, number of reps and sets, walking/running faster and longer, with possibly some incline if you are using a treadmill or elliptical. You will also use more time until you finally use up your allotted workout time. After a few more weeks, you notice that your workouts have become quite intense, and you complete your workout very tired, sweaty, and beat. **ONLY NOW, YOU ARE PREPARED** to deal with this kind of physical and mental stress. Instead of feeling overwhelmed like you will never go to the gym again, you feel good and satisfied that you completed your workout with such intensity.

In review, if you work out too intensely at first, you will build anxiety against going to the gym. This anxiety will keep you from going to the gym, just like the New Year's resolution makers. If you slowly increase the intensity of your workouts as described, you will not experience this anxiety. As your physical and mental endurance increases, you will start to feel anxiety if you don't go to the gym. Now instead of not being able to return to the gym, you cannot be kept from the gym. If you don't go to the gym, you feel great anxiety. This anxiety builds until you go to the gym. Unlike the story at the beginning of this section, this anxiety is good for you. *The stress has now flip-flopped.* Instead of not being able to force yourself back to the gym, you cannot force yourself not to go to the gym. **I CANNOT OVERSTRESS THE IMPORTANCE OF STARTING YOUR ROUTINE THE WAY I DESCRIBED.** Doing so will allow you to establish a training routine and maintain it for the rest of your life.

Diet and Exercise

DO NOT USE EXERCISE AS PART OF YOUR DIET PROGRAM. DIET IS FOR NUTRITION. EXERCISE IS FOR MUSCULOSKELETAL, CARDIOVASCULAR, AND PHYSIOLOGICAL FITNESS. You can be nutritionally fit and physically unfit, but you cannot be physically fit and nutritionally unfit. This is because your body needs nutrition to perform at any significant level physically. In any exercise or physical fitness program, whether for the average person or the extreme athlete, diet or nutrition is at least 70 to 80 percent of your success in achieving your goals. *The physical exercise provides the stress to stimulate your muscles and bones, but it is the nutrition that allows your body to repair itself and achieve new growth.*

Also, your body is designed to perform physical activity. Without being physically active, your body can malfunction in many ways. *People who are sedentary usually have lots of aches and pains in their joints and muscles.* Depending on their diet, they may have excessive carbohydrates and fats to deal with, including cholesterol and triglycerides. They correspondingly *have more problems with heart disease, high blood pressure, diabetes, fibromyalgia, and many other diseases.*

That is why **DIET AND EXERCISE** are promoted together, but they are, in reality, **TWO SEPARATE ENTITIES. THE BIGGEST FALLACY THAT CONTINUOUSLY GETS PERPETUATED IS USING EXERCISE TO LOSE WEIGHT.** Sure enough, you will use more Calories when you exercise, but it is very easy to gain weight while performing a very intense exercise program if you don't eat appropriately for your needs. Also, it is very easy to be nutritionally unfit if you don't learn to eat well. Therefore, *use exercise* to provide musculoskeletal fitness, cardiovascular fitness, and physiological fitness. *Your diet* will provide the nutrition to allow your body to achieve its maximal health. *Eating appropriately for your needs* will allow you to control your weight under any circumstances.

EXERCISE CONCLUSION

Now that you have this information, make sure you use it. **I HAVE SEEN MANY FAILURES AND FEW SUCCESSES IN ACHIEVING A LONG-TERM TRAINING ROUTINE.** Why are there so many failures with few successes? Inevitably, people get impatient with their progress. They jump into their routines with great zeal. Now they are met with the anxiety monster that I described to you. Most people are unable to cope with this monster and quit their pursuit of exercising.

YOU ARE NOW PREPARED WITH INFORMATION THAT WILL ALLOW YOU TO BE SUCCESSFUL IN ESTABLISHING AND MAINTAINING A LONG-TERM EXERCISE PROGRAM. There are variations to the information that I have presented. The initial workout times and weights I described may be an exaggeration, but some of you may need this protracted schedule to help you become successful. You may find or have used a particular approach to exercising that has helped you be successful in establishing and maintaining an exercise routine. Regardless of the approach, there is a commonality. **ALL OF THE APPROACHES KEEP THE STRESS AND ANXIETY EXPERIENCED DURING THE START-UP PERIOD TO TOLERABLE LEVELS.**

The information in the other parts of this book will help you provide your body with the best and most appropriate nutrition. **NUTRITION IS THE MOST IMPORTANT PART OF BEING HEALTHY AND BEING ABLE TO ACHIEVE A GOOD PHYSICAL CONDITION.** Just remember that regardless of how intensely you exercise, it is **UNNECESSARY TO USE ANY TYPE OF SUPPLEMENT.**

If you are unable to exercise for some reason, do the best you can.

Some physical activity will be better than none. As you age, you are going to lose some of your physical ability; that is just the way you are designed. If you do not stimulate your body enough through work or exercise, you continue to lose physical ability at a much faster rate. Eventually, you will no longer be able to walk or do many other physical activities required for daily living. Keep exercising as long and intensely as you can to avoid losing as much of your physical ability as possible.

AUTHOR'S COMMENTS

You now have **THE TRUTH ABOUT DIETS, SUPPLEMENTS, WEIGHT LOSS, AND EXERCISE. PUT THIS INFORMATION TO THE TEST.** The truth will always prevail. It may take you several years to reach your final goal, but **IT WILL NOT TAKE YOU VERY LONG TO REALIZE THAT YOU NOW HAVE THE TRUTH.** You should be able to see the fallacy in all diet programs, supplements, natural medicines, etc. *You now know that it takes a combination of nutrition, which is obtained from unprocessed or minimally processed food coupled with exercise, to achieve optimum health.* **I WISH YOU THE BEST IN YOUR PURSUIT OF HEALTH.**

Appendix 1

Classical Food Pyramid

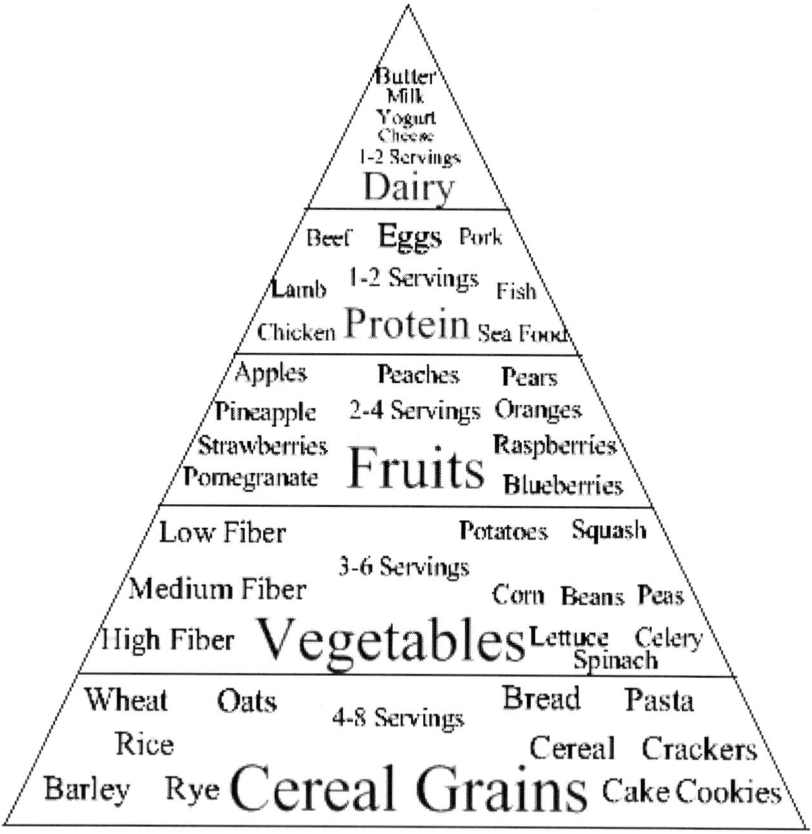

Appendix 2

New Food Pyramid

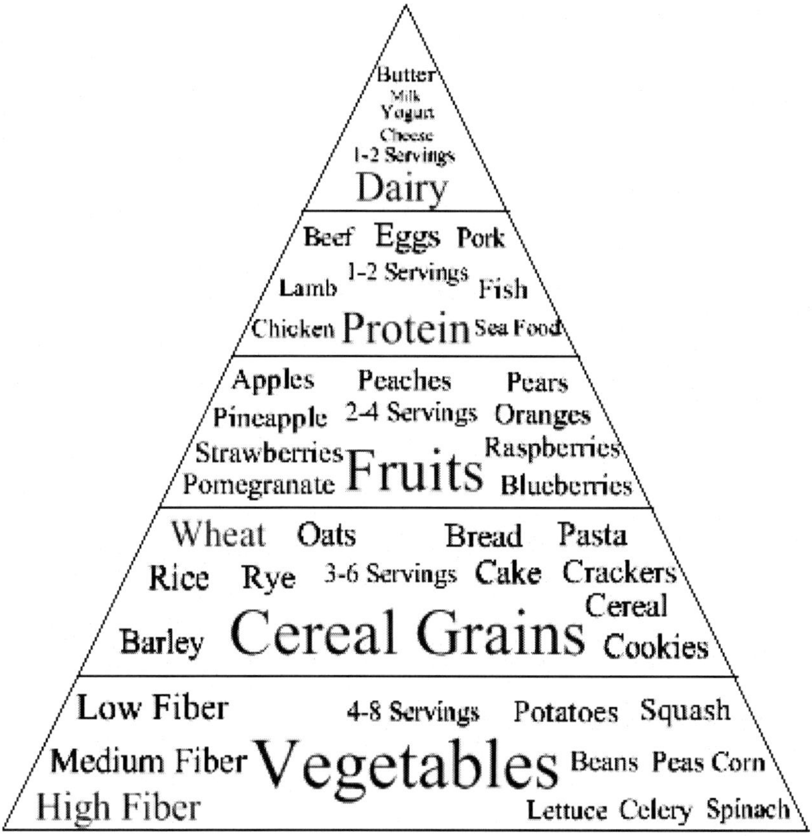

Appendix 3

Vegetarian Food Pyramid

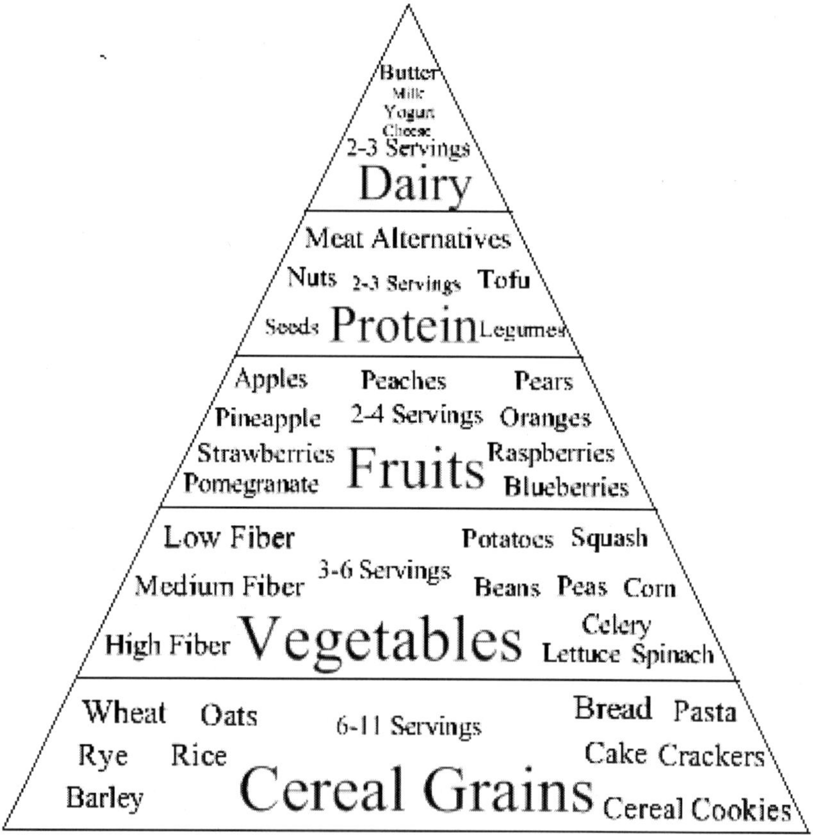

INDEX

Made in United States
North Haven, CT
04 November 2026

21765279R00113